CARING FOR THE
PARKINSON PATIENT

CARING FOR THE PARKINSON PATIENT

A Practical Guide

Edited by
J. THOMAS HUTTON, M.D., PH.D.
& RAYE LYNNE DIPPEL, PH.D.

Foreword by
Nathan Slewett, Chairman, National Parkinson Foundation

Second Edition

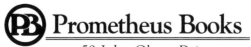

Prometheus Books
59 John Glenn Drive
Amherst, New York 14228-2197

Published 1999 by Prometheus Books

03 02 01 00   5 4 3 2

Library of Congress Cataloging-in-Publication Data

Caring for the Parkinson patient : a practical guide / edited by J. Thomas Hutton & Raye Lynne Dippel ; foreword by Nathan Slewett. — 2nd ed.
    p.   cm.
Includes bibliographical references.
ISBN 1–57392–684–1 (alk. paper)
    1. Parkinson's disease. I. Hutton, J. Thomas. II. Dippel, Raye Lynne.
RC382.C38   1999
362.1'96833—dc21   99–10843
                                                CIP

Printed in the United States of America on acid-free paper

Contents

Foreword

It is with pleasure and esteem that I recommend *Caring for the Parkinson Patient: A Practical Guide,* the Second Edition by J. Thomas Hutton, M.D., Ph.D., and Raye Lynne Dippel, Ph.D.

Dr. Hutton chairs the National Parkinson Foundation Center of Excellence in Lubbock, Texas. He is a neurologist with a Ph.D. in neuropsychology and studied under a recognized giant in the field of psychology, the late Dr. A. R. Luria. Dr. Hutton is a recognized leader in Parkinson's disease research, the psychology of Parkinson's disease, and patient care. Dr. Dippel is a psychologist. Their book emphasizes the great psychological and emotional toll of Parkinson's disease and offers novel insights into coping with these problems. To this end, they have assembled an impressive cadre of experts skilled in various aspects of Parkinson's disease.

Caring for the Parkinson Patient covers the psychological stresses of the patient, caregiver, and family in an exemplary way in the chapters "Emotional Changes in Parkinson's Disease," "Psychiatric Aspects," "Parkinson's Disease and the Family," "Parkinson's Disease and Its Impact on Sleep," "Community Support Systems," and "Caregivers Need Care, Too." This book, however, is more. There are chapters on "Diagnosis and Treatment," "Surgical Treatments for Parkinson's Disease," "Research in Parkinson's Disease," "Speech, Swallowing, and Communication," "Sexuality and Parkinson's Disease," "Nursing Aspects of Parkinson's Disease," "Cognitive Changes Associated with Parkinson's Disease," and "Occupational and Physical Therapy." There are also practical tips in the chapters entitled "Causes and Prevention of Falls in Parkinson's Disease" and "Ways to Reduce the Risk of Falling in the

Home Environment," as well as an appendix illustrating a home exercise program.

This book is one that the Parkinson patient, as well as his or her care-givers, family, friends, and physicians, should read and carry with them.

Nathan Slewett
Chairman of the Board
National Parkinson Foundation, Inc.
October 27, 1998

1

Diagnosis and Treatment

J. Thomas Hutton and Jerry L. Morris

OVERVIEW

What Is Parkinsonism?

Parkinsonism refers to a medical condition characterized by tremor, slow and reduced movements, and muscular stiffness. In the United States alone, approximately one million persons are estimated to suffer some form of parkinsonism, the most common form of which is Parkinson's disease: a slow, progressive brain disease of unknown cause affecting certain of the deeper structures (basal ganglia) in the brain. It is associated with the depletion of a brain chemical known as dopamine; this chemical loss tends to be focused particularly in a black pigmented area of the midbrain called the substantia nigra. The reduced dopamine brings about impaired communication between neurons of the substantia nigra and those of a nearby part of the brain known as the corpus striatum (the caudate and putamenal nuclei), resulting in the symptoms of Parkinson's disease (see figure 1).

Disorders that Resemble Parkinson's Disease

The symptoms of parkinsonism are often drug-induced. Tranquilizing medications are the most common drugs that cause Parkinson-like symp-

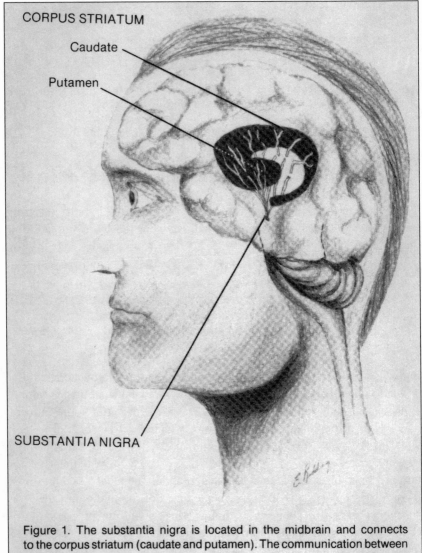

CORPUS STRIATUM

Caudate

Putamen

SUBSTANTIA NIGRA

Figure 1. The substantia nigra is located in the midbrain and connects to the corpus striatum (caudate and putamen). The communication between these structures is mediated principally by the chemical messenger dopamine.

toms. Such medications as haloperidol (Haldol), chlorpromazine (Thorazine), loxapine (Loxitane), trifluoroperazine (Stelazine), and fluphenazine (Prolixin) may give rise to clinical symptoms indistinguishable from Parkinson's disease. Reserpine, which may be used for high blood pressure or as a tranquilizing agent, also may give rise to parkinsonism. This is not to suggest that all tranquilizing medications carry such a risk factor. Tranquilizers of the benzodiazepine class—such as diazepam (Valium), chlordiazepoxide (Librium), and alprazolam (Xanax)—do not cause symptoms of parkinsonism. A gastrointestinal motility medication known as metochlopramide (Reglan) also may cause parkinsonism.

Parkinsonism can also result from small strokes that can usually be traced to a preexisting high blood pressure condition. For a person who has suffered small strokes (or lacunes), slowness of movement and stiffness of the muscles may be present in addition to general weakness or sensory loss. A careful neurological examination will usually differentiate this disorder from true Parkinson's disease. This so-called arteriosclerotic form of parkinsonism does not respond well to the medications used to treat Parkinson's disease and is more likely to be associated with medication side effects.

Encephalitis (inflammation of the brain) may also give rise to parkinsonism. A particular form of encephalitis swept the world in epidemic proportions between 1918 and 1925, leaving many persons with parkinsonism. The postencephalitic form of parkinsonism, rarely seen today, damaged the basal ganglia of the brain. Tremor was unusual with this form of parkinsonism.

In 1985, several instances of parkinsonism resulted from a street drug contaminated with a chemical known as MPTP. This extremely toxic agent selectively damages the same areas that are injured in Parkinson's disease and gives rise to the same symptoms. The victims respond favorably to levodopa, which is the principal medication used to treat parkinsonian patients. Although the discovery of MPTP was a tragedy for those afflicted, it did open up a promising new area for Parkinson's disease research (see chapter 16).

Another neurological disorder that has at times been mistaken for Parkinson's disease is essential or familial tremor. In this disorder, the hand tremor is faster and finer than that of Parkinson's disease and is most bothersome when patients attempt to use their hands. In contrast, parkinsonian tremor is slower, more coarse, and most obvious when the hands are at rest. A person with essential or familial tremor does not have muscular rigidity or slowness of movements as do parkinsonians. Essential tremor occurs sporadically, whereas the familial tremor runs in families, with approximately half the offspring developing it at some time during their lives.

Progressive supranuclear palsy (PSP) has been called a "kissing cousin" of Parkinson's disease, although it is much less frequent. It is also a progressive neurological disease that adversely affects movement, while affecting balance earlier and more severely than does Parkinson's disease. The muscular stiffness is primarily of the neck and back muscles, unlike Parkinson's disease in which extremity stiffness is observed. The diagnosis of supranuclear palsy also requires that the patient's gaze be impaired, which typically consists of an inability to elevate or lower the eyes. Memory problems are often a prominent aspect of this progressive neurological disease.

DIAGNOSIS OF PARKINSON'S DISEASE

Clinical Signs of Parkinson's Disease

As in the time of James Parkinson (1755–1824), Parkinson's disease remains a diagnosis that is established by neurological examination. Such an exam may often be sufficient to identify and exclude the other disorders just described, any of which could be mistaken for Parkinson's disease. At the present time, no readily available laboratory test exists that will confirm the diagnosis of Parkinson's disease, although the computer assisted tomography (CAT) scan and the magnetic resonance imaging (MRI) scan can rule out small strokes or tumors as causes of the parkinsonism.

The cardinal signs of Parkinson's disease are a slow resting tremor, a particular form of muscular rigidity referred to as cogwheeling (which produces rachety movements), and slow or significantly reduced movement (bradykinesia). The tremor is four to five cycles per second and most commonly observed in the hands. The tremor has been described as a "pill-rolling" type, reminiscent of the pharmacists of yesteryear who made pills by rolling them between their fingers and thumbs. Tremor may also be seen in the jaw and in the lower extremities. The muscular rigidity is usually identified by the examiner as he moves the extremities back and forth while feeling for regular jerks, as if a cogwheel were in the extremity. The bradykinesia may be of a general type, in which the person lacks the usual minor changes in position and moves slowly, or it may be noted when the person attempts rapid fine movements of the hands or feet, such as tapping the heel or opening and closing the hands.

In addition to these three cardinal signs of Parkinson's disease, a number of minor signs exist. These include changes in speech, difficulty in swallowing, the presence of drooling, a noticeably stooped posture, a lack of arm swing when walking, a shuffling gait, loss of balance, a blank staring facial expression (mask-like face), constipation, difficulty with bladder control, sexual dysfunction, and dandruff (seborrheic dermatitis). The speech pattern of a parkinsonian is that of a muffled monotone; the volume of the speech is reduced and at times may be difficult to understand. Swallowing may also be impaired with aspiration (sucking of air) occurring into the windpipe. Drooling, referred to as sialorrhea, results from lack of automatic swallowing and is aggravated by the stooped posture of those with Parkinson's disease. The lack of associated arm swing during walking represents a loss of an automatic (involuntary) movement that typically occurs when the basal ganglia portion of the brain is not functioning properly. The balance problems result from a loss of the patient's normal ability to correct changes in posture (his or her righting reflexes) and from the feet "freezing," both of which may result in serious falls. For those who have lost these righting reflexes, a slight shove may find them completely unable to regain balance. Walking consists typically of short, shuffling steps. The patient may show propulsive or retropulsive gait in which an attempt is being made to keep the feet centered beneath the body to avoid falling. Constipation, poor bladder control, and impotence point to involvement of the autonomic nervous system with Parkinson's disease.

By convention, Parkinson's disease is diagnosed when at least two of the three major signs are present, or when one major sign and at least two minor signs are identified. Few patients ever develop all the signs of the disease, and substantial variation in the symptoms are often observed. Approximately one-fifth of those with Parkinson's disease never develop tremor, so that particular component is not a requirement for the diagnosis.

Parkinson's Disease Symptoms

—slow, resting tremor
—muscular rigidity (cogwheeling)
—bradykinesia (slowness of movement)
—poor balance
—disturbance in gait (propulsive or retropulsive); "freezing" (feet immobilized suddenly)
—stooped posture
—blank facial expression
—difficulty swallowing
—reduced volume and clarity of speech
—sialorrhea (drooling)
—seborrheic dermatitis (dandruff)
—bladder control problems
—constipation
—sexual dysfunction
—mood changes
—sleep disturbance

Stages of Parkinson's Disease

Parkinson's disease is usually a slowly progressive disorder. A variety of scales have been developed to describe its severity. One commonly used clinical scale is that developed by Hoehn and Yahr, which divides the disease into five stages:

Stage I —Signs of Parkinson's disease are strictly one-sided, affecting one side of the body only.

Stage II —Signs of Parkinson's disease are bilateral but balance is not impaired.

Stage III —Signs of Parkinson's disease are bilateral and balance is impaired.

Stage IV —Parkinson's disease is functionally disabling.

Stage V —Patient is confined to bed or a wheelchair.

Progression through the stages of Parkinson's disease is highly variable. In rare instances a person may progress to stage IV or V in as little as five years, but more typically a patient may have Parkinson's disease for fifteen to twenty years before entering the severest stages. The staging of the disease also does not take into account the frequently seen clinical fluctuations. For example, an advanced parkinsonian patient may be totally bedridden (Stage V) prior to a delayed dose of levodopa, but once the medication has taken effect the patient may improve to stage II or III.

MEDICATIONS FOR PARKINSON'S DISEASE

Principles of Drug Therapy

The goal of treating Parkinson's disease with a drug regimen is to reduce functional disability. For that reason, it is important that the treating physician have an adequate knowledge of how the disease is affecting the life of each patient. A favorable balance is sought between improved motor performance and the side effects from medications. For example, a surgeon, a seamstress, or a typist will have more need to maintain tight control of the disease and will likely risk more medication side effects than would, say, an inactive or retired person. A good general rule of treatment is to improve everyday activity, not to eradicate every sign of parkinsonism. With the exception of the first few years of levodopa treatment, it is usually impractical to mask completely the signs of the disease. Attempts to do so are fraught with increased risks of medication side effects.

A person with Parkinson's disease who is well versed in the goals and the possible adverse aspects of treatment and who understands the expected course of the disorder can greatly enhance the therapeutic outcome. The treating physician, who is often a neurologist, will have knowledge about which aspects of the disease are likely to improve with a given medication and what side effects are most likely to occur. An awareness of the expected progression of the disease is also important. Too often patients incorrectly assume that worsening motor function is a result of ineffective medication rather than a sign identifying the changing nature of their disease. An evolving clinical picture requires periodic checkups and dosage readjustments.

Good and open communication between patient and treating physician is important. Patients bring to this relationship knowledge about the impact that the disease has had on their lives and a set of values that speak to the degree of risk and disability that can be tolerated. For their part, physicians bring medical and scientific knowledge about the disease and a general understanding of how other patients in similar circumstances have responded. The doctor/patient relationship is in a very real sense a contract requiring both to do their best to assure the most favorable outcome.

Patients who are knowledgeable about Parkinson's disease and have a good grasp of the symptoms provide the possibility of limited flexible dosage schedules. From time to time these individuals may need increased medication—for example, prior to physical exertion or just before making a public appearance. It is useful for physicians to provide dosage flexibility for such persons in order to tailor the drug therapy to their needs. On the other hand, some patients present who ostensibly are unable to tolerate any antiparkinsonian medications. In each of these instances, however, the person had invariably failed to recognize that the "side effects" were in fact the signs of the disease itself. Dosage flexibility is only practical with a well-informed patient. Except for emergencies, it is desirable for the patient to check with the doctor prior to discontinuing medications.

Anticholinergic Agents (tremor medications)

The first effective treatment for Parkinson's disease was tincture of belladonna (atropine and hyoscine) and was introduced in the nineteenth century by the famous French neurologist Jean Martin Charcot (1825–1893). A large number of other anticholinergic and antihistaminic medications were introduced during the 1940s and 1950s. These agents are most useful for the treatment of tremor. Since tremor is frequently the first sign of Parkinson's disease, it is not at all surprising that the anticholinergic and antihistaminic agents are often the first medications used in the treatment process (see table 1). The anticholinergic agents also dry the mouth and may therefore prove useful in treating drooling. Unfortunately, this class of medication has little or no positive effect on rigidity, slowness of movement, or other features of Parkinson's disease. The anticholinergic agents are of value in treating drug-induced parkinsonism and postencephalitic parkinsonism.

A time-honored, if slightly outmoded, clinical concept describes an imbalance between the cholinergic system and the dopaminergic system in the brains of parkinsonians. This concept suggests that the symptoms of the disease may be improved either by increasing the amount of dopamine in the brain or by reducing the amount of acetylcholine (see figure 2). The anticholinergic medications interfere with brain acetylcholine transmission and are believed to create a better balance between these two principal brain chemicals. Those anticholinergic agents still commonly in use include trihexyphenidyl (Artane), benztropine (Cogentin), biperiden (Akineton), and procyclidine (Kemadrin).

Anticholinergic medications may give rise to side effects. For example, constipation and difficulty with emptying the bladder may result. Bladder problems and constipation are fairly common among parkinsonian patients in any case, but these conditions can be further aggravated if anticholinergic agents are part of the treatment. Blurring of vision and confusion may result from the anticholinergic effect on both the eyes and the brain. Anticholinergic agents also impede sweating, which could lead to heat exhaustion for patients in hot climates or during the summer months. On the other hand, some Parkinson's disease patients experience excessive and abnormal sweating, which may be reduced by the anticholinergic medications.

TABLE 1

MEDICATIONS COMMONLY USED IN THE TREATMENT OF PARKINSON'S DISEASE

MEDICATION	STAGE	DOSAGE	BENEFITS	MAIN SIDE EFFECTS
Anticholinergics:				
Trihexyphenidyl (Artane)	mild-moderate	2-20 mg/day	Reduces tremor, drooling	Mental changes
Benztropine (Cogentin)	mild-moderate	0.5-6 mg/day	Reduces tremor, drooling	Constipation
Biperiden (Akineton)	mild-moderate	2 mg/day	Reduces rigidity (especially in drug-induced PD)	Difficulty emptying bladder
Procyclidine (Kemadrin)	mild-moderate	2.5-15 mg/day	Reduces rigidity (especially in drug-induced PD)	Dry mouth
Antihistamines:				
Diphenhydramine (Benadryl)	mild-moderate	25-200 mg/day	Reduces tremor; mildly sedating	Drowsiness
Chlorphenoxamine (Phenoxene)	mild-moderate	50-300 mg/day	Reduces tremor; mildly sedating	Drowsiness
Amantadine (Symmetrel)	mild-moderate	100-300 mg/day	Helps slowness, stiffness, tremor	Visual hallucinations, confusion, dizziness
Levodopa (Sinemet)	all stages	100-1000 mg/day	Helps slowness, stiffness, tremor	Nausea, confusion, postural dizziness, dyskinesias
Selegiline (Eldepryl)	mild-moderate	5-10 mg/day	Mild benefit for slowness, stiffness, tremor	G.I. upset, sleeplessness
Dopamine Agonists:				
Bromocriptine (Parlodel)	all stages	1.25-20 mg/day	Helps slowness, stiffness, tremor	Confusion, postural dizziness
Pergolide (Permax)	all stages	0.75-6 mg/day	Helps slowness, stiffness, tremor	Confusion, postural dizziness
Pramipexole (Mirapex)	all stages	1.5-6 mg/day	Helps slowness, stiffness, tremor	Confusion, postural dizziness
Ropinirole (Requip)	all stages	3-24 mg/day	Helps slowness, stiffness, tremor	Confusion, postural dizziness
Apomorphine	severe	4-10 mg/dose	Rescue therapy	G.I. upset, confusion, penile erection
Cabergoline (Cabaser)	all stages	0.5-15 mg/day	Helps slowness, stiffness, tremor	Confusion, postural dizziness
COMT Inhibitors:				
Tolcapone (Tasmar)	moderate-severe	300 mg/day	Helps slowness, stiffness, tremor	Liver failure, dyskinesias, urine discoloration, diarrhea
Entacapone (Comtan)	all stages	200 mg with each levodopa dose	Helps slowness, stiffness, tremor	Dyskinesias, diarrhea

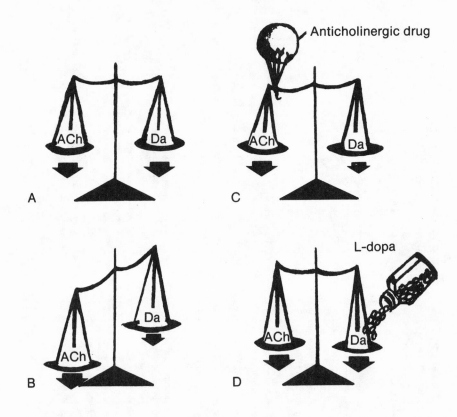

Figure 2. This figure demonstrates the balances between acetylcholine (ACh) and dopamine (Da) for normal and parkinsonian states. Panel A demonstrates the normal balance between acetylcholine and dopamine in normal, healthy persons. In B, which represents Parkinson's disease, the deficiency of dopamine is represented by an imbalance in favor of acetylcholine. Panel C represents restoration of this balance by an anticholinergic drug, which effectively reduces the effect of brain acetylcholine. Panel D represents an alternative therapeutic strategy of restoring the balance by providing levodopa, which is converted to dopamine, thereby increasing brain dopamine levels.

Antihistamines

Antihistamines are a category of medications closely related to anticholinergics. It may be that the pharmacologic benefits of the antihistaminic agents result from anticholinergic properties, so that the antihistamines are generally considered along with the anticholinergic agents. The antiparkinsonian effects of the antihistamine medication is clearly unrelated to their effects on histamine.

Diphenhydramine (Benadryl) is an over-the-counter agent that is used particularly for the treatment of tremor. This agent has less risk of causing or aggravating bladder and bowel problems, but may give rise to drowsiness, especially in the first few weeks of use.

Amantadine (Symmetrel)

Amantadine may be an initial treatment for Parkinson's disease, especially if slowness of movement or rigidity are the principal symptoms. It is generally well tolerated and acts clinically like a weak form of levodopa. The precise mechanism of action is unknown. It may exert its antiparkinsonian effect by increasing the release of dopamine stored in the brain. Amantadine does have a beneficial effect on rigidity, slowness of movement, and tremor.

The discovery of the antiparkinsonian effect of amantadine was serendipitous. Dr. R. S. Schwab learned from a patient who had been prescribed amantadine for influenza that her Parkinson's disease was helped. Dr. Schwab subsequently confirmed this observation—patients looked better and felt better when taking amantadine. This agent is now commonly used for mild and moderate forms of the disease.

Some experts believe that the wholesome effects of amantadine may be short-lived. Others believe that the effect is ongoing, yet the progression of the disease after several months requires the physician to substitute or add a stronger medication. Whether or not the effects of amantadine are ephemeral, discontinuation of the medication may be associated with a substantial increase in parkinsonian symptoms. Restarting the medication will usually reestablish control at the level that was present prior to discontinuance. If amantadine is to be discontinued, it is best to taper the dosage downward prior to discontinuing.

Visual hallucinations are a disturbing side effect of amantadine; they are observed particularly in advanced Parkinson's disease. The hallucinations frequently take the form of nonthreatening people or animals and may be very realistic. This adverse effect will go away when the medication is discontinued. Livido reticularis is a purplish skin mottling of the legs that may also result from treatment with amantadine. This skin reaction is not serious but usually prompts discontinuation of the medication. Other possible side effects include congestive heart failure, lightheadedness or faintness upon standing, and swelling of the ankles. Visual blurring, constipation, and difficulty emptying the bladder may also occur as side effects of amantadine.

Selegiline (Eldepryl, Carbex)

Selegiline is a selective inhibitor of monoamine oxidase type B (MAO-B). It was initially developed and marketed as a neuroprotector. There was some evidence that it could slow the underlying progression of Parkinson's disease. Unfortunately, further evaluation has not been able to clearly document a neuroprotective benefit of selegiline. Nevertheless, it does seem clear that it provides at least a mild beneficial effect on parkinsonian symptoms. For this reason, it may be useful early in the disease, particularly before levodopa is needed.

Levodopa (Sinemet, Madopar)

The introduction of levodopa (also called L-Dopa) in the mid-1960s for the treatment of Parkinson's disease followed the important discovery that dopamine was reduced in certain brain structures in parkinsonians. Replacement therapy with levodopa, which is converted in the body to dopamine, brought about many dramatic clinical improvements. Levodopa continues to be the most widely used agent in treatment regimens and is effective at all stages of the disease. Typically, levodopa therapy is begun when muscular rigidity or slowness of movement starts to impair everyday performance significantly. This is a highly effective treatment for the symptoms and signs of Parkinson's disease, but neither levodopa nor any other antiparkinsonian agent has yet to affect a slowing of the underlying disease.

To prevent rapid breakdown of levodopa in the body, the drug is combined with either carbidopa or benserazide. Carbidopa/levodopa (Sinemet) is marketed throughout North America and Europe, while benserazide/levodopa (Madopar) is marketed throughout Europe and Canada. By using either carbidopa or benserazide as blocking agents to prevent breakdown of levodopa before it reaches the brain, the total required amount of levodopa is reduced by 80 to 90 percent.

When a person with Parkinson's disease starts treatment with Sinemet or Madopar, the effects are typically dramatic. The bradykinesia (slowed or reduced movement), rigidity, and tremor are greatly improved to the extent that the person may be almost unaware of parkinsonian symptoms. This so-called "levodopa honeymoon" usually lasts from two to five years. During this period of time, the patient usually does not feel any wearing off of the medication. Nevertheless, many parkinsonians eventually begin to experience the "wearing-off" phenomenon or "end of dose" failure.

Wearing-off phenomenon may occur subtly: for example, when a person awakens in the morning and finds that the symptoms of the disease are particularly prominent. The patient may also experience the return of symptoms prior to the next scheduled dose of levodopa. At this point in the treatment the patient can usually sense when the medication "kicks in," and becomes acutely aware of the need to take the medication regularly.

The scientific understanding of the wearing-off phenomenon and the on/off syndrome is incomplete. The wearing-off phenomenon probably results from reduced storage of dopamine throughout the basal ganglia so that controlling the signs of the disease requires a fairly stable level of levodopa in the bloodstream. Unfortunately, the blood level of levodopa is short-lived, lasting only a few hours.

There are three general approaches to treatment once the wearing-off phenomenon sets in. The traditional approach is to take standard Sinemet or Madopar at more frequent intervals, often in smaller doses. A second approach is to change to one of the controlled-release forms of these medications that were introduced in the early 1990s. This approach springs from the observation that levodopa, when infused intravenously at a constant rate, will largely stop motor fluctuations. The development of Sinemet CR and Madopar HBS were based on this finding. The third general approach to aid in controlling wearing-off is to add another agent, typically a dopaminergic agonist or COMT inhibitor.

Although levodopa is the drug of choice for most parkinsonians, it is not without side effects. When beginning the medication, it is best to start with small doses and build up over a period of several weeks. A positive effect will usually be seen in four to five days, but the complete effect may take several weeks. The slowly increased dosage will also limit nausea. Vomiting occurs occasionally, but it is rarely so severe as to prevent continued use of the medication. When beginning levodopa, it is best to take it with food. Later, as tolerance is developed and more complete absorption is needed, the drug may be taken on an empty stomach or with a light nonprotein snack. (Dietary considerations will be discussed in more detail in this chapter and in chapter 6.)

With long-term use of levodopa, drug-induced abnormal movements may occur (dyskinesias). These movements may consist of mouth or tongue movements, or quick, nonpurposeful movements of the extremities. At times, writhing movements or fixed abnormal postures of the hands or feet may occur. These drug-induced dyskinesias usually occur when the levodopa in the bloodstream is at its maximum ("on" dyskinesia), although occasionally they occur when the drug level is at its minimum in the blood ("off" dystonia). Dyskinesias are usually seen in the context of advanced disease, suggesting that the underlying brain substrate is important in the evolution of this side effect. In addition, the long-term effects of levodopa bring about a change in the dopamine receptors in the brain, which may be involved in the evolution of dyskinesias.

Mental confusion and hallucinations pose a growing problem not only for the parkinsonian patient but for the treating physician as well. In 1817, when James Parkinson originally described the mental aspects of the disorder now bearing his name, he referred to "the senses and intellect being uninjured." It is likely that prior to the advent of levodopa, persons with Parkinson's disease did not survive long enough for parkinsonian dementia to occur. In addition, it is now well recognized that most of the antiparkinsonian agents may give rise to confusion. This aspect of parkinsonism is particularly perplexing to treat. As a general rule, if a state of confusion is experienced, all antiparkinsonian medications are discontinued with the exception of minimal doses of levodopa. The relative benefits of the drug must be weighed against its side effects. At times a drug holiday may be tried to determine if the confusion disorder is indeed the result of medication. Drug holidays, nevertheless, are not without significant risk of severe immobility with aspiration pneumonia and pulmonary emboli.

Lightheadedness and fainting can be side effects of levodopa. Upon arising quickly, the blood may rush to the legs, thus depriving the brain of adequate blood supply. Although this may occur in patients who are not treated with levodopa, it is often worsened by the medication. Typically, this is not so severe as to alter therapy, but at times it may require the wearing of elastic stockings or, if necessary, discontinuing levodopa.

When taking levodopa, it is essential that non-selective monoamine oxidase (MAO) inhibitors not be taken. This should not be confused with the antiparkinsonian drug selegiline (Eldepryl), which is a *selective* inhibitor of MAO type B. The non-selective inhibitors (such as Parnate, Eutonyl, Furoxone, Marplan, and Nardil) are rarely prescribed today, but for a period of time they were used to treat depression. Such a combination has the potential to cause severe elevations in blood pressure and pulse rate. Alpha methyl dopa (Aldomet), which is used to treat high blood pressure, should not be prescribed in combination with levodopa as it reduces the effect of levodopa much like the major tranquilizers described earlier.

Dopamine Agonists

In contrast to levodopa, which is converted to dopamine in the substantia nigra that in turn secondarily stimulates the corpus striatum (caudate and putamenal nuclei), a dopamine agonist directly stimulates the dopamine receptors in the corpus striatum. The agonist agent in effect fools the corpus striatum into accepting it as dopamine.

Although dopamine agonist agents may be used alone, they are typically added to the medication regimen when levodopa begins to lose its effectiveness. Dopamine agonists can be beneficial in smoothing out the daily course of motor fluctuations seen with levodopa-treated Parkinson's disease. The addition of a dopamine agonist to levodopa will allow smaller amounts of the latter to be used, which may offer some theoretical advantage. Some neurologists believe that this may be of some benefit in forestalling the onset of motor fluctuations. In this country, bromocriptine (Parlodel) and pergolide (Permax) have been available for many years. Two new agonist agents, pramipexole (Mirapex) and ropinirole (Requip), became available in the United States in 1997.

Cabergoline (Cabaser) is a new agonist agent that is not marketed for Parkinson's disease in the United States, but it is available for this indication in Europe and elsewhere. Another new dopamine agonist, referred to as N-0923 TDS, is in clinical testing in the United States at this time. N-0923 TDS is novel in that the medication is delivered through a transdermal delivery system (or skin patch). Sustained delivery of the dopamine agonist through the skin patch offers several theoretical advantages compared to dosing by mouth, and the results of initial clinical testing of N-0923 TDS are encouraging. Apomorphine and lisuride are older agonist agents that are also available in other countries, but not in the United States. Interestingly, apomorphine is currently being studied in clinical trials in this country as "rescue" therapy for patients with severe motor fluctuations.

Bromocriptine (Parlodel)

Bromocriptine (Parlodel) was the first dopamine receptor agonist agent available for treating Parkinson's disease and it is still used widely. It is most effective in the early to middle phases of the disease, although it is usually reserved for the middle stages. Bromocriptine is almost as effective as levodopa in treating bradykinesia, muscular stiffness, and tremor, but it is most effective when used in combination with levodopa. Bromocriptine needs to be started in low doses, then gradually increased over a period of several months to lessen the risk of side effects. Although patience is required to use this medicine, the recipient is rewarded with improved motor function.

Bromocriptine has significant potential side effects, one of the most disturbing of which is confusion. Confusion has been observed in nearly half the patients who use this therapy, but is most prominent in patients with advanced disease. Confusion is much less likely when the agent is used in the early stages of Parkinson's disease and when used in younger patients. The severity of the confusion episode is greater than that associated with levodopa, amantadine, or the anticholinergics. Whereas a mild dementia may occur with Parkinson's disease, caution is advised when using bromocriptine for these patients. The drug-induced confusion disorder subsides over several days when the medication is discontinued. Nausea, vomiting, and lightheadedness are other side effects of bromocriptine. Dyskinesias have also been described, but they are less common with bromocriptine than with levodopa.

Pergolide (Permax)

Like bromocriptine, pergolide is derived from ergotamine and can be expected to have similar side effects. The major difference between bromocriptine and pergolide is in the profile of dopamine receptors stimulated. Whereas bromocriptine stimulates D_2 receptors and inhibits D_1 receptors, pergolide stimulates both D_1 and D_2 receptors. This profile has theoretical advantages and may provide improved symptomatic effect. It is worthwhile to note that levodopa (Sinemet), the "gold standard" in therapy for Parkinson's disease, is also active at both types of receptors.

Pramipexole (Mirapex)

Pramipexole is one of two nonergoline agonists approved by the U.S. Food and Drug Administration in 1997. It improves motor function, reduces length and severity of "off" time, and allows for reduced levodopa dosing. The side effects of pramipexole are primarily dopaminergic (i.e., similar to that seen with Sinemet); there may be increased dyskinesias, hallucinations, nausea, constipation, and insomnia. Treatment with pramipexole avoids the ergot-related side effects associated with bromocriptine and pergolide. Most noteworthy, symptomatic orthostatic hypotension is uncommon with pramipexole.

Pramipexole must be started at a very low dose and increased gradually over several weeks to reach the best therapeutic effect. It is generally taken three times a day. The maximum recommended dose is 2.0 mg three times daily.

Ropinirole (Requip)

Ropinirole is the other nonergoline dopamine agonist agent that has recently been approved by the FDA for treating Parkinson's disease. The beneficial effect on parkinsonian symptoms and the side effect profile are very similar to pramipexole.

Ropinirole also must be started at a low dose and increased gradually to obtain the maximum beneficial effect. Dosing is typically three times a day. The maximum recommended dose is 8.0 mg three times daily. This increased range of therapeutic dosing compared to pramipexole may be advantageous for some patients.

COMT Inhibitors

Catechol-O-methyltransferase (COMT) metabolizes or breaks down dopamine and levodopa, the active agent in Sinemet, into an inactive metabolite. Reducing the amount of COMT in the body would be useful for parkinsonian patients treated with Sinemet in that more levodopa could be delivered to the brain. Medications known as COMT inhibitors have been developed recently for just this purpose. These agents inhibit COMT in the body, thus increasing the bioavailability and transport of levodopa across the blood-brain barrier. They are always used along with levodopa. Tolcapone (Tasmar) is available at this time in the U.S., and entacapone (Comtan) is still in clinical testing.

Tolcapone (Tasmar) inhibits COMT peripherally (outside the brain) and has some central (within the brain) inhibitory effect at high doses. It extends the length of the clinical response to levodopa (Sinemet), improves motor function, and is beneficial for motor fluctuations. Since it increases the availability of levodopa, the side effects are primarily dopaminergic (similar to Sinemet). These include new or increased dyskinesias (unintended movements), nausea, and hallucinations. Approximately 8 percent of tolcapone-treated patients develop diarrhea. Usually, this can be controlled with over-the-counter diarrhea remedies, although occasionally it can be severe and can lead to dehydration. The typical dose of tolcapone is 100 mg taken three times a day. It is not uncommon to have to reduce the dosage of levodopa due to dyskinesias. At the time of this writing, new safety concerns have just been announced. Several persons taking tolcapone have developed fulminating hepatitis and have died. Rigorous blood tests are recommended should tolcapone be used. Additional information will likely be forthcoming.

Entacapone (Comtan) is undergoing clinical testing and is not marketed at this time. It inhibits COMT only in the periphery. It also increases the bioavailability of levodopa, prolongs the clinical response to levodopa, and improves motor fluctuations. The side effects seen with entacapone are primarily dopaminergic in nature (e.g., dyskinesias and nausea). Like tolcapone, diarrhea is a possible side effect. Entacapone is usually given along with each dose of levodopa (Sinemet). As with tolcapone, treatment with entacapone often necessitates reducing the dosage of levodopa due to dyskinesias.

Antidepressant Medications

Depression occurs in 20 to 40 percent of parkinsonians, although in most cases it is mild. The origin of the depression results from Parkinson-related brain chemical changes, but psychological reactions to the chronic illness also play a part (see chapter 4).

Commonly used antidepressant medications for depression in Parkinson's disease include amitriptyline (Elavil), imipramine (Tofranil), doxepin (Sinequan), and nortriptyline (Pamelor). Antidepressant effects may not be realized for one to three weeks. All of these medications can cause drying of the mouth, increased constipation, and difficulty emptying the bladder.

A newer class of antidepressant medications, called selective serotonin re-uptake inhibitors, is now available and offers faster onset and fewer side effects. Agents in this class include Prozac, Wellbutrin, Effexor, and Paxil.

OTHER THERAPEUTIC APPROACHES

Exercise

Exercise plays a valuable role in the overall treatment plan. A regular program of exercise assists in maintaining muscle flexibility and will even reduce the need for medication. Stretching exercises are particularly beneficial given the increased muscular rigidity found in parkinsonian patients. Consultation with a physical therapist can be useful to define an appropriate group of exercises that may be continued at home (see chapter 7).

Diet

In general, changes in diet have little effect on Parkinson's disease. At times, however, especially in advanced stages of the disease, protein may impair the transport of levodopa to the brain. In such instances, in which parkinsonians tend to go "off" following a protein meal, a protein redistribution diet may prove helpful. The concept of protein redistribution is not to decrease the overall amount of protein in the diet, but rather to redistribute dietary protein to a time when the patient is likely to be sedentary or asleep. Typically, protein redistribution moves the protein to the evening meal, while breakfast and lunch are high in carbohydrates, fruits, and vegetables (see table 2).

At times when advanced parkinsonians are having dyskinesias, ingestion of a protein snack may be of benefit; by impairing levodopa transport it thus diminishes the levodopa-induced dyskinesias. Such a protein snack may also be of some benefit in counteracting levodopa-induced vivid dreaming and nightmares.

Vitamin B_6 is known to inhibit the effectiveness of levodopa. This effect is seen only when levodopa is taken without an inhibitor, so that no particular concern exists when a parkinsonian patient is taking either Sinemet or Madopar. Nevertheless, if levodopa is being taken in the form of Larodopa, then multiple vitamins containing vitamin B_6 should be avoided. Should vitamin supplements be desired, then a vitamin preparation without B_6 should be prescribed (such as Larobec).

Diets high in fiber and fruit may also help to reduce or avoid constipation. For additional dietary information see chapter 6.

TABLE 2

PROTEIN REDISTRIBUTION DIET FOR PARKINSONIANS*

DAYTIME (PRIOR TO 5:00 P.M.)	EVENING MEAL
An unrestricted quantity of the following foods can be consumed [less than 10 gms. (grams) of protein]:	Meal should contain Recommended Daily Allowance for individual's age at ideal weight (approximately 30-50 gms. after 10 gms. consumed during day.

Fluids:	Coffee, tea, soda (nondiet), all fruit and vegetable juices, water, nondairy liquid creamers (e.g., Polyrich).
Fruits:	All fresh and dried fruits.
Vegetables:	All green and yellow vegetables (lettuce, onions, cucumbers, cauliflower, broccoli, squash, carrots, etc.); potatoes (skinless) cooked any way, including french fries.
Breads & Cereals:	Certain cereals that are low in protein (Rainbow Brite, Rice Krispies, and Rice Chex—should contain 2 gm. or less protein per serving).
	Graham crackers, melba toast, fried onion rings, toaster pastries.
Desserts:	Italian ice, sherbet
Condiments:	Oil, vinegar, margarine, butter, herbs, spices, sugar, honey, jellies and jams, pickles, hard candies, mints, powdered nondairy creamers.

FOODS TO AVOID BEFORE 5:00 P.M.:

Meat, meat products, fish, egg whites (yolk contains no protein), gelatin, dairy products (milk, sour cream, cheeses, yogurt, cottage cheese, ice cream); legumes such as kidney beans, lima beans, soy or pinto beans; nuts, peanut butter, chocolate, cookies, cakes, pastry, or pizza.

*Adapted from "Influence of Dietary Protein on Motor Fluctuations in Parkinson's Disease," by Jonathan H. Pincus, M.D., and Kathryn Barry, M.S.N., R.N. *Archives of Neurology* 44 (1987):270–272.

SUPPORT ACTIVITIES

Parkinson's disease can be frightening for both the patient and the family. Access to a variety of support activities can assist those afflicted and their families to adjust to this chronic disease. The treating physician may be able to provide answers to many questions and can also offer referrals to a variety of health care professionals for such additional needs as physical therapy, occupational therapy, speech therapy, social services, dietary consultation, or long-term counseling. Support groups and information and education centers may provide practical and useful information about coping with Parkinson's disease in a comfortable environment. All of these areas are discussed in the chapters that follow.

SUGGESTED READING

Duvoisin, Roger C. (1985). *Parkinson's Disease: A Guide for Patient and Family.* New York: Raven Press.

Pincus, Jonathan H., and Kathryn Barry. (1987). "Influence of dietary protein on motor fluctuations in Parkinson's disease." *Archives of Neurology* 44:270–72.

2

Emotional Changes in Parkinson's Disease

Matthew E. Lambert

Although it was originally described as primarily involving motor abnormalities and fluctuations, over the past several decades considerable research has shown that numerous cognitive, sensory, perceptual, and emotional changes often accompany Parkinson's disease (PD). It has been estimated that between 30 to 50 percent of PD patients suffer depression or anxiety symptoms some time during the course of their disease. Some symptoms may be mild and inconvenient, while others may be so severe as to require formal mental health treatment.

Early explanations of emotional reactions in PD patients emphasized the disability and lifestyle changes that caused patients to become despondent and fearful. This was consistent with emotional reactions experienced by patients suffering other chronic illnesses, who experienced difficulty coping with changes resulting from the illness itself. Yet PD patients were found to suffer significantly higher rates of emotional disturbance than other patients with chronic illnesses. Subsequent research demonstrated that neurotransmitter deficits in the brain chemicals serotonin and norepinephrine, linked to depression and anxiety disorders, tended to occur more often in PD patients.

Although there seems to be a significant relationship between neurotransmitter deficits and emotional reactions in PD patients, the role of stress and coping difficulties cannot be excluded. It is most likely that a combination of these two factors contribute to the actual manifestation of depression or anxiety. As a result, the PD caregiver is helped by understanding how depression and anxiety are manifested and the treatments that are available.

DEPRESSION

According to the fourth edition of the American Psychiatric Association's *Diagnostic and Statistical Manual of Mental Disorders* (DSM-IV), depressive disorders involve several diagnostic categories. Diagnoses often associated with depression in PD include Major Depressive Disorder, Dysthymic Disorder, Adjustment Disorder with Depressed Mood, and Mood Disorder Associated with a General Medical Condition. By far, the most common depression diagnoses given to PD patients are Major Depressive Disorder and Mood Disorder Associated with a General Medical Condition. These disorders, however, may be easily misdiagnosed or underdiagnosed, since many symptoms characteristic for PD overlap with those necessary to make the depression diagnosis.

The DSM-IV requires five of nine symptoms to be present for a two-week period for a diagnosis of a significant depressive episode to be made. These symptoms include: depressed mood, as indicated by either subjective report or observation by others; diminished interest or pleasure in everyday activities; significant weight loss or weight gain; insomnia or hypersomnia; psychomotor agitation or retardation; fatigue or loss of energy; feelings of worthlessness; diminished ability to think or concentrate; and recurrent thoughts of death or suicide. As can easily be seen, many of these symptoms are common to the overt manifestations of PD. The masked faces characteristic of PD often obscure sad facial expressions or other overt appearances of depression, while weight loss and sleep difficulties are common to PD. Tremor or dyskinesia can be confused with psychomotor agitation, as the latter often worsens to the former. And the cognitive difficulties experienced in PD may interfere with the detection of similar deficits that are depression-induced. Thus, it may be difficult at times to distinguish between those symptoms reflective of an actual depressive experience and those characteristic of PD itself.

In detecting PD depression, greater reliance may need to be made on the specific symptoms associated with depression. Unprecipitated tearfulness or crying, low self-esteem and vocalized self-deprecation, feelings of hopelessness and helplessness, and irritability are symptoms often seen in depression and not specifically characteristic of PD. The presence of these symptoms may distinguish the true underlying emotional state from that discerned by direct observation only. Similarly, recurrent thoughts of death and suicide or suicide attempts are more commonly associated with a true depressive disorder than PD alone. Any of these symptoms being present should alert the caregiver to the presence of a concomitant depressive disorder and the need for treatment. When there is uncertainty over the presence of a depressive disorder, referral to a mental-health specialist familiar with PD depression can help to eliminate any remaining diagnostic uncertainty.

PD DEPRESSION TREATMENT

Once depression is identified, it is essential that treatment be undertaken since the depressive symptoms themselves may magnify and exacerbate PD symptoms. Recent research has demonstrated that depressive symptoms may further impair fine-motor performance. Additionally, cognitive deficits associated with PD may be magnified by the cognitive symptoms of depression. Compliance with medication or physical-therapy regimens may also be problematic, as motivation may wax and wane with cycles in a depressive syndrome. Overall, depression can adversely affect almost all aspects of PD.

Since depression in PD is primarily related to changes in neurotransmitter chemicals, pharmacological treatment may be the most effective intervention. Antidepressant treatment is discussed elsewhere in this volume and will not be reviewed here. Nevertheless, pharmacological treatment may be significantly enhanced by psychological intervention designed to help patients cope more effectively with limitations caused by their disease and to enhance their quality of life. Psychological intervention provided by a psychologist or other mental-health professional should focus on helping the PD patient maintain mastery over as many parts of their lives as possible. Such mastery experiences could include maintaining physical activity, social involvement, and mental stimulation. When previously enjoyable activities are no longer possible, efforts can be made to find new activities equally rewarding and interesting as those rendered unattainable by PD symptoms. Moreover, psychological intervention can help to alter negative self-perceptions that may arise as functional ability declines and the need for caregivers increases.

It is important to note, however, that psychological intervention does not need an extended period of time to be effective. Significant changes can usually occur within six to eight treatment sessions held on a weekly basis. In most cases, Medicare and supplemental insurance policies will cover almost all the cost for such treatment.

ANXIETY

Although depressive symptoms have received the greatest attention in PD, it has been increasingly noted that many Parkinson's patients suffer significant anxiety symptoms, either with or without concomitant depressive symptoms. Moreover, previous research has indicated that many Parkinson's patients suffer significant anxiety prior to the onset of their motor symptoms. This has raised the question whether anxiety may actually be either a predisposing factor or a precursor to PD. Whatever the answer, anxiety symptoms play a significant role in managing medications, functional ability, and overall quality of life for the PD patient.

The etiology to anxiety symptoms in PD, however, is much less certain than it is with respect to depression. Neurotransmitter changes, similar to those noted as the basis for depressive symptoms, have been implicated for anxiety as well. It has also been noted that PD dopaminergic therapy may produce anxiety reactions in many patients. Fear of falling, choking, or being unable to control motor behavior in social situations can also produce significant anxiety reactions and behavioral changes. Again, it is unlikely that there is one single cause for anxiety in PD patients; rather, it is likely to be a combination of medical and psychological factors.

Regardless of their basis, anxiety reactions do occur quite frequently in the PD patient. In one study, approximately one-third of the PD patients surveyed met the criteria for an anxiety disorder listed in the DSM-IV. Anxiety disorders commonly diagnosed in PD patients include Panic Disorder, Social Phobia, and Generalized Anxiety Disorder. It is also likely that a significantly greater number of PD patients suffer milder anxiety reactions that are not of sufficient severity to warrant an anxiety disorder diagnosis, but that still impact PD symptoms and management. A survey conducted in our research center revealed that approximately 72 percent of the PD patients who responded experienced anxiety to some degree, and 33 percent indicated that they suffered anxiety *before* their PD was diagnosed. Mild anxiety was noted to involve physical, cognitive, and behavioral symptoms which may or may not overlap with their neurological disease's manifestations. PD patients reported dizziness, arm or leg numbness, shortness of breath, wobbly or rubbery legs, tingling in the fingertips, having a lump in the throat, and feeling disoriented and confused. Cognitive anxiety symptoms also noted related to fear of passing out, losing control, having a heart attack, babbling or talking funny, or screaming. Because these mild anxiety symptoms have been noted in many patients, we have now started to refer to their presence as the Parkinson's Anxiety Syndrome.

Although anxiety is by definition an undesirable state, its effect on PD only serves to magnify this distress by worsening motor and cognitive symptoms of the disease. Anxiety produces changes in heart rate, breathing, blood pressure, muscle tension, body temperature, and stomach activity, all which are manifestations of autonomic arousal. These symptoms are part of the "fight or flight syndrome" and are produced by increased levels of the neurotransmitter chemical norepinephrine. As autonomic arousal increases, there is a magnification of symptoms already present due to PD. Tremor, freezing, rigidity, and dyskinesias can all become more pronounced as the autonomic arousal from anxiety amplifies them. This produces a greater risk of falling during freezing episodes, since freezing may be prolonged more than usual. Furthermore, behaviors performed easily during relaxed states can be rendered impossible and frustrating by worsened motor functioning when anxious. "Off" periods can also be magnified, with fluctuating anxiety levels making it difficult to manage dosage and timing of antiparkinsonian medications. Racing and disjointed thoughts precipitated by anxiety can also give the appearance of greater confusion and cognitive impairment. And, as anxiety becomes more commonplace for the PD patient, it creates still more anxiety and a vicious circle of both increased anxiety and increased motor/cognitive impairment.

PD ANXIETY TREATMENT

Since the etiology of anxiety in PD is less certain than for PD-related depression, treatment options are more diverse. Both pharmacological and psychological treatments may be effective, and decisions regarding their use vary according to the specific anxiety symptoms present, their severity, and responses to treatment efforts. Pharmacological treatment of PD anxiety in many ways mirrors the treatment for depression. Several antidepressant medications have demonstrated significant efficacy for treating such anxiety problems as Panic Disorder, Social Phobia, and Generalized Anxiety Disorder. (Again, the interested reader is referred to the chapter on pharmacological depression treatment in this volume for a full discussion of such medications.) Additionally, more traditional anti-anxiety medications, such as the benzodiazepines, can be used to reduce anxiety symptoms, whether mild or severe in nature. However, side-effects from either antidepressant or anti-anxiety medications may pose problems for some PD patients. Antidepressants known as Selective Serotonin Re-uptake Inhibitors (SSRIs) may produce paradoxical responses of sleep disruption, increased anxiety, and tremor which can worsen PD symptoms. Certain benzodiazepines have also been contraindicated for some patients as their pharmacological effects may worsen PD symptoms. Medications may also enhance drowsiness and cause clouding of consciousness, which are especially undesirable for the PD patient. Many times, if such adverse reactions are experienced, a shift in medication to a similar one in the same class may produce the desired benefits but without the unwanted side effects. Unfortunately, this is often a trial-and-error process, with the effects of a specific medication on any particular patient being unknown until it is tried.

Then, too, anxiety symptoms may not be of sufficient severity to warrant pharmacological intervention; or patients may not be able to tolerate antidepressant or anti-anxiety medications due to side effects; or there may be a desire to minimize the use of any medications other than those specifically needed for PD treatment. In these cases and others, psychological interventions are available which do not pose the potential problems often seen with medications. Psychological interventions have also been demonstrated to be highly successful and as effective as medication in treating a wide variety of anxiety problems and disorders (i.e., Panic Disorder, Social Phobia, and Generalized Anxiety Disorder). These treatments emphasize teaching patients to develop control over their physiological and cognitive symptoms of anxiety, along with applying those control skills in situations where anxiety occurs. Typically, a combination of relaxation training and cognitive restructuring techniques are taught during weekly individual or group counseling sessions, with homework assignments given to practice these techniques in anxiety-producing situations. With practice, some patients can also control the PD symptoms associated with heightened anxiety and the fears or worries that trigger anxiety states.

The rest of this chapter presents a psychological treatment model currently in use to help PD patients learn to control anxiety symptoms. This treatment program is completed over an eight-week period, with hourly treatment sessions held once a week.

SESSION 1: DIAPHRAGMATIC BREATHING TREATMENT

Diaphragmatic Breathing Rationale

Anxiety produces numerous changes in autonomic physical functioning: heart rate, blood pressure, breathing pattern, body temperature, stomach activity, muscle tension, and so on. As part of this process, the neurotransmitter chemical norepinephrine is secreted, which also has effects on other body functions, including a patient's PD symptoms. Increased tremors, freezing, swallowing problems, falling, and others symptoms can all occur as the result of anxiety. This makes management of PD medications more difficult as anxiety may counter their beneficial effects, which only makes the patient's quality of life less positive. Because of this, efforts to control anxiety are essential to the overall management of PD.

Diaphragmatic breathing is one method that can be used to reduce physical symptoms of anxiety and their effects on PD. Slow, deep breathing helps return the body to a more relaxed state by slowing heart rate, lowering blood pressure, reducing stomach activity, lowering body temperature, and reducing muscle tension. This then helps to reduce the pressure put on tremor, freezing, falling, and other PD symptoms.

Diaphragmatic Breathing Instruction

Get into a comfortable position, either sitting or lying down, and close your eyes. Try to let your breathing get into a slow, rhythmic pattern without the pressure to breathe too quickly or too slowly. Let your body's own natural rhythm take over. It is often helpful to say the word "CALM" slowly to yourself each time you breathe out. As you practice the relaxation exercise, try to relax various muscle groups in your body, starting with your head and working down to your feet. Spend about a minute or two relaxing each muscle group before starting with the next group. A good sequence for the muscle groups would be: head and upper neck, neck and upper shoulders, shoulders and arms, chest and upper back, abdomen and lower back, hips and upper legs, and lower legs and feet.

Remember that relaxation is an acquired skill, just like learning to drive a car. The more you do it, the better you get. It is recommended you practice twice a day for at least 20 minutes. Also, try and practice

about the same time every day, with the second relaxation session just
before bed.

SESSION 2: COPING WITH "OFF" STATES AND FREEZING

Diaphragmatic Breathing During "Off" or "Freezing" Rationale

As noted, anxiety involves numerous physical symptoms related to heart
rate, breathing, muscle tension, stomach activity, and so on. Anxiety also
worsens tremors, freezing, swallowing, risk of falling, and other PD
symptoms. Greater problems with PD symptoms only add to the anxiety
already experienced, further reinforcing it and making control of PD
symptoms more difficult. As you have been learning over the past week,
diaphragmatic breathing can be used to reduce anxiety and its physical
symptoms. Also, while practicing the relaxation activity over the past
week, you probably noticed that tremors and rigidity might have been
lessened during that time. Because of this, diaphragmatic breathing may
be used to help ease and facilitate management of the PD symptoms of
tremor, rigidity, and falling during "off" states or when freezing occurs.
Practicing relaxation during "off" times or when PD medications are
wearing off can help minimize symptoms until the next medication dose
is taken. Additionally, should freezing occur, it tends to cause anxiety and
fear of falling. By using relaxation when freezing, an end to the freezing
episode may be brought about more quickly, reducing the chance of
falling and immobility.

Diaphragmatic Breathing Instruction

Continue to practice the diaphragmatic breathing relaxation exercise used
during the past week twice daily. As you become better at using the relaxation exercise, try to use it during "off" states or before taking your next
dose of PD medications to help ease the motor symptoms that worsen
during those times. Also, during any episodes of freezing, try slowing
your breathing down and relaxing before trying to move further. Once
you feel more relaxed, then try moving again.

SESSION 3: CONTROLLING ANXIETY BEFORE IT IS A PROBLEM

Recognizing Anxiety Building and Controlling It Earlier

Anxiety builds over time, and often the full anxiety picture will not arise during freezing episodes or "off" states. As anxiety builds, PD symptoms tend to worsen until the anxiety is out of control. Once anxiety builds to its peak, it is difficult to turn it back down. Often, various parts of the body can provide clues that anxiety is building. Learning to recognize anxiety as it builds and controlling it earlier in the process can help keep anxiety from getting out of control. It is important, then, to practice controlling anxiety as it builds and learning to turn it back down. The difficult part, of course, is that once you start waiting for anxiety to come, it often does not appear like it is supposed to. You can simulate anxiety, however, by using what you have already learned about breathing. If anxiety is reduced by diaphragmatic breathing, an opposite or rapid and shallow breathing pattern could bring about anxiety-like symptoms and make PD symptoms worse. You can use such a breathing technique to bring about physical symptoms of anxiety so that you can then practice controlling anxiety as it builds. Alternating rapid and shallow breathing with diaphragmatic breathing will help you recognize anxiety symptoms as they build and then control them before they get out of hand. The key is to practice bringing on anxiety and then turning it off again and again in non-stressful and safe situations. Later, you can practice using this strategy to learn how to control anxiety in stressful situations or where PD symptoms cause particular problems.

Rapid Breathing–Anxiety Induction Instruction

When you have slowed down your breathing to bring about a feeling of relaxation, you can use the reverse to bring about anxiety. Again, get yourself into a comfortable position and relax. You may find that two or three minutes of diaphragmatic breathing is all that is needed to relax yourself now. First, notice how your body feels in the relaxed state. Now breathe rapidly for 30 seconds, similar to how a dog would breathe if it were panting. Pay attention to the physical changes that occur while breathing this way. Then use diaphragmatic breathing to control anxiety for the next 2 minutes. Contrast the physical sensations between the fast breathing and the relaxed breathing. Repeat the rapid breathing for about 1 minute, followed again by the relaxation breathing exercise to control anxiety for 2 minutes. Again, focus on and contrast the physical sensations experienced during each type of breathing. Repeat rapid breathing again for 2 minutes, followed by the relaxation breathing exercise to control anxiety for 4 minutes. Notice the physical sensations each time.

Remember, relaxation is an acquired skill and so is learning to control anxiety. The more you do it, the better you get. It is recommended you practice the alternating anxiety induction and relaxation exercises, as described above, before doing the full diaphragmatic breathing exercise twice daily. During each series of exercises, focus on the changes occurring in your body to determine when anxiety is building. Additionally, use relaxation when necessary 20 to 30 minutes before taking each dose of medication or during episodes of freezing. Furthermore, note when anxiety begins to build during the day and try and turn it back down when you feel it grow.

SESSION 4: CONTROLLING ANXIETY IN DIFFERENT SITUATIONS

Generalizing Anxiety-Control Strategies to Problem Situations

As you learn to control anxiety that is building or during freezing or "off" times, you can start to use these skills to control anxiety in other situations. Imagery is one way to learn to control anxiety in specific situations. This is done by imagining what it would be like to experience and cope with situational anxiety and its behavioral effects while actually in safe and protected settings. Once these coping skills are mastered, they can be transferred to those real-life anxiety-producing situations. To start this process, create a list of situations where anxiety has interfered with your activities or worsened your PD symptoms. Try to come up with about 5 to 10 different situations that vary in the amount of anxiety they produce. Then order the situations from least distressing to most distressing according to the amount of anxiety they cause. A helpful way to do this is to assign each situation a number value from 10 to 100, with 10 being only minimally distressing and 100 being overwhelmingly distressing.

Once the list is developed, you can start to practice experiencing and then controlling anxiety in each situation, using the anxiety-induction technique while imagining what it is like to be in that situation. Start with mastering the least distressing situations and work your way up to the most distressing ones.

Imaginal Exposure with Anxiety-Induction Instruction

While sitting comfortably, imagine what it feels like to be in the situation that has caused anxiety while practicing the anxiety-induction procedure. During the anxiety induction, notice how the various parts of your body feel. Try to remember how your body felt the last time you actually were in that situation and had anxiety problems. Continue the anxiety induction for 1 minute, followed by the diaphragmatic breathing exercise to control anxiety for 2 minutes, while feeling what it is like physically to control the anxiety in the situation and overcome it. Repeat this imaginal exercise with anxiety induction again for 2 minutes, followed again by diaphragmatic breathing to control anxiety for 4 minutes along with imagery of coping in the situation. Be sure to imagine *what your body actually feels like* in the situation, rather than simply trying to see yourself in the situation. During each series of alternating breathing exercises, focus on the changes occurring in your body to determine when anxiety is building. Practice this alternating pattern of anxiety induction and anxiety control at least three times for each situation on your list along with your regular relaxation practice. Once the situation can be imagined without anxiety building, then move on to the next situation on your list until all the situations have been mastered.

SESSIONS 5-8: CONTINUED RELAXATION PRACTICE

Generalizing Anxiety-Control Strategies to Problem Situations

Anxiety-producing situations come up all the time, and so it is necessary to practice controlling anxiety in any new situations that may arise. When new situations come up, add them to your list of distressing situations and practice controlling them as you have before. Order them according to the severity of the anxiety associated with them. Practice controlling the anxiety three times for each situation or until it is under control. When you feel you can overcome the anxiety associated with the situation, then attempt to apply the technique in the real-life situation. Remember, after practicing the alternating breathing for anxiety induction and relaxation, practice the full relaxation exercise for about 20 minutes. Additionally, use relaxation when necessary before taking each dose of medication or during episodes of freezing. Furthermore, note when anxiety begins to build during the day and try to turn it back when you feel it grow. As anxiety-producing situations occur, continue to add them to the list as appropriate. Keep practicing these techniques daily. Making them a part of your lifestyle helps to keep anxiety from getting a foothold again and makes overall management of your PD symptoms easier.

Coping with Worries and Fears

Often, it is worries or fears about worsening symptoms, embarrassment, loss of ability, and so on which precipitate anxiety and cause the worsened functioning that is of so much concern. These worries and fears stem from the values and beliefs people have about themselves and how others will view them. Because this is often a significant factor in the PD patient's anxiety, it is addressed as part of each treatment session along with the more formal relaxation and coping skills training. This process is often referred to as Cognitive Restructuring.

Cognitive Restructuring Rationale

Although physical symptoms of anxiety tend to be the basis for worsening PD symptoms, this does not explain why some people find certain situations anxiety-provoking and others do not. In many cases, it is the beliefs that people have about themselves, their behavior, and how others perceive them that influence their emotional reactions. High self-expectations help motivate people to work harder, while low expectations provide little incentive at all. But when high expectations are not met, frustration tends to set in, while negative expectations can set up situations where self-fulfilling prophecies occur. For example, the fear of being unable to move or shaking in public may only serve to increase physical anxiety and actively create the feared situation, which then reinforces those expectations. This will lead to general feelings of failure rather than success.

To deal with this dilemma, patients need to learn to be more realistic in their expectations for themselves and others, which may involve changing some of their underlying values and beliefs. This can be done by changing some of the things that patients say to themselves that reflect their expectations, values, and beliefs. By changing these "self-statements," some of the stress that patients put on themselves can be reduced, thereby reducing anxiety and its untoward effects on PD symptoms.

The first thing that you must do is to look at the things you say to yourself that could be causing anxiety. Examples of such self-statements include: "I have to be in control all the time"; "People are talking about my walking and shaking"; or "I'm not as good as I used to be because of my Parkinson's." It is easy to see how these statements are reflections of individual values and beliefs. Moreover, these statements can actually interfere with performance and lead to increased anxiety levels. They are often referred to as "maladaptive cognitions" because they interfere with coping and mastery over life events. And because they are reflections of deeply held values and beliefs, most people are unaware that they are even saying them to themselves, making them "automatic thoughts." Moreover, these maladaptive cognitions, these automatic thoughts, are really people making predictions and interpretations about themselves and others. It is by this process that anxiety builds in different situations and leads to worsened functioning.

To change maladaptive cognitions and reduce the anxiety caused by them, you have to work at identifying and challenging your beliefs in order to give yourself flexibility in dealing with PD and other problems. Ask yourself, for example, *"How good am I at predicting the future?" "Where is the evidence to support my beliefs?" "Can I read other peoples' minds?" "What other explanations are there?"* Keeping written information about maladaptive cognitions is also quite helpful.

Cognitive Restructuring Practice

Changing beliefs, worries, expectations, and fears is not easy; it requires practice. Once again, the more you do it, the better you get. It is often helpful to keep track of the thoughts that cause anxiety and practice changing them to more rational thoughts. Writing down negative self-statements that produce anxiety when they occur can also be very helpful. This can be done in a notebook or on a pad of paper. If you have problems writing, ask a spouse, family member, or other caregiver to write them down for you. Asking that person to prompt you to think about your self-statements can be a good substitute.

Whatever method you use for keeping track of maladaptive cognitions, it is important to focus on the fears, worries, expectations, values, or beliefs that form the basis for your self-statements. Pay particular attention to thoughts that occur during situations in which PD symptoms are leading to increased anxiety. As you record your maladaptive cognitions, begin the process of challenging them by writing alternative or more realistic statements just below them. Also practice saying the more realistic statement to yourself out loud. Practice this each time you start getting anxious in a certain situation or when anxiety is making your PD symptoms worse. It is also helpful to practice repeating more realistic self-statements while doing the relaxation exercise in anxiety-producing situations. This associates positive self-statements and coping with physical feelings of relaxation and control over anxiety.

The more you practice this, the easier it will get. If you keep practicing each time you start noticing anxiety, then this will be come part of your normal style for coping with anxiety and stress.

Seeking Professional Help

If the PD patient or caregiver is uncertain about the presence of depression, anxiety, or some other emotional problem associated with the disease or how to treat it, seeking help from a qualified mental health professional is important. Mental health professionals include psychiatrists, clinical psychologists, social workers, psychiatric nurses, and licensed professional counselors, among others. Many of these specialists have expertise in treating the emotional problems associated with PD. When seeking a specific mental health professional, it is important to determine if the professional has experience working with the emotional problems stemming from PD, as not all may have the required expertise. A few simple questions can often help determine a professional's experience with PD, and caregivers should not be shy in asking those questions. If you need help in finding an experienced mental health professional, try asking your neurologist or family physician. Once an appropriate mental health professional has been identified, effective treatment can produce positive results in a very short time.

3

Parkinson's Disease and the Family

Karen Boyd Worley and Raye Lynne Dippel

When an individual suffers from Parkinson's disease, it is not just a personal matter but a reality that affects every member of the family. Parkinson's disease taxes the family's financial, physical, and emotional resources. The uncertainty and doubt prior to diagnosis, the crisis of diagnosis, the hardship of new symptoms and setbacks, and for some the heartbreaking necessity of nursing home care combine to test a family's coping skills. At times, family members rise above the difficulties and demonstrate not only adequate adjustment but also inspiring personal growth. On other occasions, the stress becomes too much and families begin to behave in dysfunctional ways.

All families are clearly challenged by the presence of Parkinson's disease in a loved one. What accounts for the ability of some families to struggle through hard times—to form uniquely workable solutions to their situation—while others seem to become mired in unpleasant, hurtful, or unhealthy interactions? Why do certain families find themselves able to cope well at some times and poorly at others? While there are no hard and fast rules to account for the complex and unique workings of any individual family, systems theory offers a way of looking at how families interact and can help professionals in their efforts to facilitate a family's move beyond unpleasant or unhealthy situations.

DEPRESSION, COGNITIVE IMPAIRMENT, AND THE FAMILY

The Parkinson's disease symptoms in which family influence may be particularly important are depression and cognitive impairment. The beneficial effects of levodopa, so helpful for motor symptoms, are of no use in alleviating these two secondary complaints. Between 30 and 40 percent of all parkinsonian patients have shown low levels of depression, but these are consistently higher than other comparison groups, healthy or ill. It is apparent in many cases that when an individual patient responds positively to levodopa, thus reducing physical symptoms and increasing ability to be active, depression decreases. In this situation, *hope* for maintaining gains may be as important as an increased activity level. Recent research (Wallhagen and Brod, 1997) suggests that both the patient's and the caregiver's sense of well-being is elevated if they perceive that they have the ability to control day-to-day symptoms. The caregivers reported feeling less burdened if they perceived that they had some control over the severity of the symptoms. Interestingly, the perceived level of control the patient or caregiver felt over the progression of the disease did not appear to affect the level of well-being or the level of burden. Parkinson patients and their caregivers may understand that ultimately there is no cure for Parkinson's disease; however, the belief that they can make a difference in the day-to-day management of the disease may reduce their sense of helplessness.

Considering the progressive nature of the disease, it is no wonder that a diagnosis of parkinsonism can have a profound emotional effect on patients and their loved ones. This gives support to the notion that the depression associated with the disease is not entirely physiologically based. The positive or negative adjustment of patients and their families to this situation is often closely related. In fact, the importance of viewing the caregiver/care receiver relationship as a mutual, interconnecting dyad is critical. Both patient and family members have profound abilities to influence each other in negative or positive ways. In a study of caregivers of geriatric patients, it was found that the mood of the care receiver was related to the mood of the caregiver (Drinka, Smith, and Drinka, 1987). Similarly, other investigators have found that the quality of the relationship between the caregiver and the care receiver was related to lower levels of key types of caregiver strain after hospital discharge (Archbold, Stewart, Greenlick, and Harvath, 1990), and that a better relationship quality with a dependent parent was associated to less caregiver-perceived burden and less family conflict (Manne and Zautra, 1989).

The positive or negative adjustment of patients and their families to the illness is often closely related to the patient's level of depression, which in itself can be a life-threatening disease. As many as half of all parkinsonian patients suffer from depression, compared to only 10 percent of the general population. Although the depression that parkinsonian patients suffer is typically mild, a significant number report moderate to severe depression and report levels of depression greater than other groups of patients who suffer from the chronic and irreversible motor impairment, such as that brought on by arthritis. Many individuals with Parkinson's disease are greatly frustrated by the rigidity, akinesia, and tremor that interfere with their ability to complete even the most simple task, whether it be buttoning a shirt or writing a check. When the ability to move from place to place is made difficult, individuals may restrict their social activity, thereby intensifying feelings of loneliness and isolation. Parkinsonian patients report embarrassment at their tremor, their shuffling gait, and their poor posture. The frustration that a patient feels may express itself as the appearance of being irritable, demanding, or excessively dependent. These behaviors put stress on marital and family relationships. The guilt associated with placing extra burdens on family members tends to lower the patient's self-esteem. If the patient's activities are severely restricted, it may necessitate early retirement along with the accompanying financial worries.

New activities must be developed to prevent the onset of boredom. The fear experienced when contemplating an unknown future or personal mortality must be faced head on. Long-term sorrow, persisting past the initial diagnosis when medical personnel are generally most available for support, has been identified in a significant proportion of couples and families faced with the day-to-day reality of this disease (Hainsworth, Eakes, and Burke, 1994; Lindgren, 1996). Caregivers and care receivers have noted that sorrow appears to be triggered by loss of future plans, restricted social life, and inability to travel and participate in hobbies.

Besides the emotional impact of the disease and the requirements of caregiving, other problems—problems not necessarily related to Parkinson's disease but more to other types of life events or the typical challenges of advancing age—can contribute to depression. These may include the death of family members or friends, family conflict, financial or career difficulties, or other psychosocial stressors. Given that parkinsonian patients may have a biological propensity toward the development of depression besides the stressors just discussed, it is important that the physician, nurse, psychologist, or family members recognize signs of depression and act to treat the disorder. This is also true for the caregiver. Besides being painful, clinical depression may greatly impede the ability of the caregiver to continue providing the day-to day-care and encouragement that patients require.

The family may have an indirect impact on the patient's level of cognitive impairment. Between 20 and 30 percent of parkinsonian patients have cognitive impairments serious enough to cause significant difficulty in their lives. Even more—perhaps the majority—report some decline in their mental capacities. But, like depression, there are other factors in a patient's life that may contribute to cognitive impairment. For example, typical Parkinson symptoms such as the mask-like face, soft, slurred speech, and difficulty maneuvering all contribute to social isolation and apathy. Certainly, as patients become more isolated and apathetic, environmental stimulation is significantly diminished. This lack of stimulation contributes to the likelihood of depression and decreased intellectual stimulation, which in turn can cause an existing cognitive impairment to appear even more serious than it is.

It is important to caution families and professionals alike that the presence of depression or cognitive impairment does not automatically indicate a problem in the care that a particular family is giving or in the attitude with which the care is given. These are both common symptoms of the disease that do not respond to typical Parkinson drug therapy, such as levodopa. Depression and its related cognitive impairment, however, does respond to antidepressant medications, which can be prescribed by a physician.

THE MYTH OF THE NORMAL FAMILY

The myth of the normal family suggests that such a family does not experience stress. With that definition, it would certainly be a challenge to find even one temporarily "normal" family. A typical fairy-tale ending to a love story is "and so they got married and lived happily ever after." As anyone with a family knows, this is when the trouble just begins! Salvador Minuchin, a major contributor to the concept of structural family therapy, describes the myth of placid normality in a family without stress as just that—a myth. Certainly the presence of Parkinson's disease exacerbates whatever stress is present. By way of illustration, a man who has had an ongoing conflict with his mother-in-law is not likely to have a miraculous new love and appreciation for her just because she has developed Parkinson's disease. Instead, the "normal" level of stress generated between mother-in-law and son-in-law may increase to disruptive proportions as involvement between the two families changes due to the disease.

FAMILY SYSTEMS

Family systems theory can provide guidelines for evaluation and treatment intervention without necessarily creating a special category for the family that does its best to cope with a difficult situation. Systems "theory" is the result of the rather unremarkable observation that people are influenced by others and by the way they interact with one another. Several key ideas in systems theory will be discussed, including: (1) having a *structure* that must constantly undergo transformation; (2) undergoing specific *stages* of development that require restructuring; and (3) needing to *adapt to changed circumstances* to maintain continuity and enhance the social growth of each member.

Structure

The structure of a family may be explained by defining subsystems of functional groups of members. These subsystems may be formed according to age, function, sex, or other factors. For example, the spouse subsystem consists of the husband and wife. It serves as a refuge for the couple and is a source of authority in the family. The sibling subsystem gives a child an opportunity to learn skills in negotiating and competing with other children. Subsystems that cross generational boundaries may include a parent, a grandparent, and/or a child. In a well-functioning family, the subsystems have clear but flexible boundaries. Parents have a strong alliance in which they support each other and do not allow the children to mediate problems that are appropriately handled by themselves. Likewise, a healthy adult family does not allow the parents to mediate all problems between siblings.

When Parkinson's disease strikes a person at the top of the family hierarchy, it can throw the whole family structure into disarray. In many families, the adult children may rigidly cling to the familiar authority patterns. Together with the ill parent, the children may conspire to deny the severity of symptoms in order to preserve the authority of the family patriarch or matriarch. In such a situation, appropriate care may not be provided. While continuing to provide needed respect for the head of the family, some "role reversal" would be appropriate. The children may need to help care for the parent rather than the other way around. For example, an aged mother with Parkinson's disease may insist on continuing to cook a large Thanksgiving dinner for the entire family, despite the fact that she suffers from emotional stress and physical strain. Her children could offer to host the dinner or contribute to the cooking and cleaning. It is important, however, not to rob individuals with physical limitations of opportunities to assist and participate (albeit moderately) in all their usual activities. Responsibilities may shift but personal dignity must never be ignored.

Stages of Development

Familial structure reveals a great deal about a family at a given point in time, but not necessarily how the family changes over time. According to a number of therapists and theorists, most families progress through predictable stages in their group life cycle. Each stage is initiated by a particular life event that requires change and adjustment by every family member. One of the family's basic tasks is to integrate stability and change so that the unit, as well as each of its individual members, can grow without becoming stuck or overwhelmed by sudden, drastic changes. Each stage presents the family with specific tasks that must be mastered. The traditional stages that a family passes through are: (1) courtship; (2) marriage and becoming a couple; (3) childbirth and young children; (4) middle marriage with school-age children; (5) late middle age when the children begin leaving home; and (6) old age. There are typical problematic patterns which indicate that the family is not handling new changes. Poor resolution at any one stage makes resolution at later stages more difficult. The most common types of stage-related problems are normal, acute stage-specific difficulties; maladaptive responses to the specific pressures of a given stage; and chronic problems related to unresolved issues from some prior developmental stage(s).

Members of the typical family may be at different stages, which further complicates family systems. For instance, a family consisting of a husband and wife may have several grown children in varying stages of leaving home, getting married, or having their own children. The parents of this couple may be in the stage of "old age" with complications that leave them more dependent on their children. This husband-and-wife subsystem may not only have the responsibility of caring for their own children (and probably their grandchildren), but their parents as well.

Families who get "stuck" in one of these stages may find it difficult to function effectively. By example, John and Ellen, a late-middle-age couple, had four children (see figure 1). The youngest had limited intelligence and learning disabilities that resulted in delayed emotional and

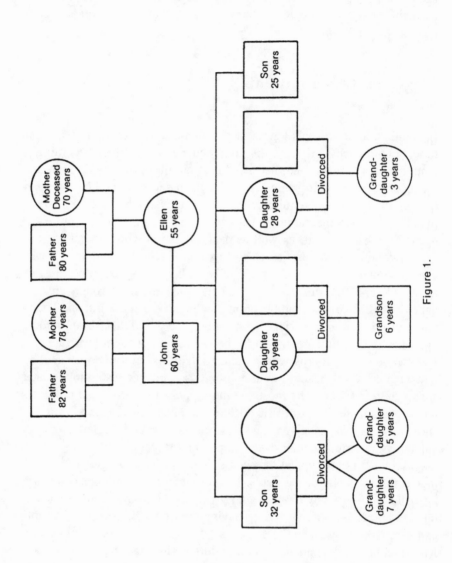

Figure 1.

cognitive maturity. This twenty-five-year-old son was routinely unemployed and living at home. The three other children, who had moved out of the home, had gone through divorces or other crises, and during the last seven years one or more of them had moved back into the home temporarily. In addition, John and Ellen had assumed important responsibilities for the daily care of their grandchildren. Clearly, this family was finding it difficult to move successfully through the stage of "children leaving home."

Both John and Ellen had major health complications of their own. Ellen had recently undergone successful treatment for cancer. Both John and Ellen worked full time. The family was obviously experiencing multiple stressors that John and Ellen were attempting to mediate. As might be expected, such stressors resulted in several levels of conflict—marital, parent-child, and sibling. In addition, Ellen's father, a widower, developed Parkinson's disease and mild dementia, which rendered him unable to care for himself. He had always lived nearby and depended on his daughter for assistance in managing his home. All family members "assumed" that Ellen would care for him.

Through trial and error, this family made adjustments that encouraged successful movement through the stage of "children leaving home," resulting in less stress and greater independence for all family members. The children were encouraged to reside outside of the home, and the parents were more realistic about what they were capable of doing for their children. An apartment was built in the back of the house to allow Ellen's father more independence and privacy in a safe environment, one in which he would benefit from frequent family interaction. This offered John and Ellen greater opportunities to have their "alone" times, during which they would go on frequent weekend trips, thereby reducing the stress brought on by family members always "asking" for assistance. The children had grown to be very dependent on their parents for help in a wide variety of ways, from unstopping the commode to watching the grandchildren, sewing a new dress, making a loan, and so on. With gentle encouragement, the children learned to rely on themselves or to find others in the community to assist them with their projects. Ellen's brother and sister were also invited to play a greater role in the care of their father. Although these adjustments were initially difficult to make, the family has generally resolved the stage of "children leaving home" and a much calmer, more loving family atmosphere exists.

The following case history illustrates how one couple coped with the diagnosis and development of Parkinson's disease as they entered the stage of "retirement and old age." Martha and George had been married for many years when Martha was diagnosed with Parkinson's disease. For several weeks she relied heavily on the support of her minister as she struggled to find the courage to tell her husband. Martha's fears were well founded; George was devastated by the news. He remembered the effect that Parkinson's disease had on a relative and her family at a time well before the advent of effective drug therapy. George saw his hopes for a comfortable retirement dashed. Of even greater importance were his concerns for Martha's well-being. Somehow, George and Martha clung together as they tried to comfort one another in this time of overwhelming confusion and sadness. Now, years later, Martha is at a good level of adjustment in the course of her illness. She and George have worked out an "optimal" regimen of diet, exercise, social activity, and scheduling of medication which allows Martha several hours of rewarding activity per day. The couple emphasizes "flexibility" as their most important policy in reducing stress. Although George is the identified caregiver in the relationship, he notes the tremendous emotional support he gets from his wife. He gratefully points out her strength and support when he suffered a heart attack a few years ago.

These are just a few examples of how the inherently complicated tasks of normal life stages can become even more difficult to move through when a family member has Parkinson's disease. In such situations, short-term family therapy with a mental health professional experienced in family counseling and familiar with the special problems of Parkinson's disease may be helpful. Such assistance may foster reorganization of resources and hasten movement through the tasks at hand.

ADAPTING TO CHANGED CIRCUMSTANCES

A family is subjected not only to inner pressure from developmental changes in its members and subsystems, but also from outer pressures that may result from problems one or more family members may have with work, school, the law, the economy, or any of a number of outside influences. Integral to the process of change and continuity that the family must accomplish is accommodating to new situations constantly presented by family members and the community. While all families must cope with these changes, more serious problems arise when families increase the rigidity of their relationship patterns and boundaries in response to stress and avoid or resist exploration of any alternatives.

An example of this is the case of Mary and Herbert, who had mutually agreed that Herbert was head of the household and breadwinner, while Mary was the homemaker and cook. Both had stringent expectations for an immaculate household and regular home-cooked meals. As Mary became progressively more disabled with Parkinson's disease, it became more difficult for her to live up to this standard. She voiced her complaints to friends and relatives, but not to her husband. Herbert did not understand how hurt and disappointed Mary was at her perception of his lack of support in her time of need. This stress exacerbated her symptoms. Both became more and more frustrated, irritable, and depressed, making it more difficult to bridge the widening gap between them. Herbert interpreted his wife's increasing difficulty in performing everyday activities as malingering, which he resented. As communication became tenser and less productive, even simple solutions—such as hiring someone to help around the house or occasionally allowing family members to bring in food—could not lessen the resentment between Herbert and Mary. While early intervention by a mental health professional probably would not have changed their long-held beliefs about the roles that men and women were expected to fulfill in marriage, it might have allowed Herbert and Mary to come to grips with her illness, to communicate with one another directly when problems needed to be solved, and to recognize their need for each other's support in a time of difficult transition.

Rigid boundaries erected by husbands and wives sometimes cause them not to let any "outsiders" help. David and Elaine kept David's illness a secret even from their grown children for a number of years after the initial diagnosis of Parkinson's disease. This effectively barred the children from providing help for their father and mother, both of whom had health problems. Elaine performed her duties so well that her husband became increasingly passive, dependent, and fragile. After Elaine's death, the children and a live-in companion allowed David to remain successfully in his own home. Despite grief over his wife's death, David has been able to take a stronger hand in directing his own medical care and daily activities. In this situation, it was Elaine's unfortunate death that was instrumental in loosening up the boundaries and allowing help from family and support from a live-in companion to come in and strengthen David's contacts with the outside world. A sensitive recognition of Elaine's hovering care by a concerned health professional could have helped to encourage the beneficial use of family members and community resources before her death, thus aiding this couple's adaptation to changing circumstances.

FAMILY INTERVENTION

How do families know when they are "stuck," and how do they find professional guidance to adapt to the increasing demands of caregiving? The following example illustrates how one family had been relatively successful during the "children leaving home" stage until their mother, Mrs. Smith, developed Parkinson's disease. The adult children, now married and enjoying thriving relationships with their own spouses and children, became very concerned and anxious about their mother's fragile appearance and her diminished ability to manage her own affairs. She had always been a fiercely independent professional woman who managed on her own.

As the disease progressed, the family members came under increasing stress. The oldest son, Don, who lived several hundred miles away, began booking frequent trips home to arrange for his mother's care and to maintain the company she owned. These added duties put considerable stress on his marriage and limited the time he could spend with his young children. Conflicts soon arose between the adult children. For example, the older siblings were angered by the continued demands that their youngest brother, Kenny, made on their mother. His siblings had always resented the relatively few restrictions placed on their "baby" brother during his formative years. As a child, he typically eluded punishment for infractions of rules and generally got whatever he wanted. The youngest brother's current lack of sensitivity to his mother's needs and limitations infuriated the other siblings, who not only argued with him but found themselves confronting their mother, who defended him. These conflicts increased the family's stress levels and presented strong roadblocks to successful group problem-solving and adjustment.

This situation is consistent with the many caregivers who note conflict with other family members over caregiving activities. Strawbridge and Wallhagen (1991) noted that 40 percent of the caregivers that they surveyed communicated a relatively serious family conflict, usually with a sibling who was not providing assistance at the level the caregiver expected. Caregivers in this study had significantly higher levels of perceived burden and poorer mental health than did caregivers who reported low levels of family conflict, even when the quality of the caregiver's relationship with the parent, the extent of caregiver tasks, and income, gender, and age were taken into account. In the previous example, long-tolerated conflicts were exacerbated by the demands of caregiving for the mother.

What the family may consider a no-win situation can benefit from a careful assessment. A list of questions was developed by Remnet (1979) to assist families in examining their interactions and to assess their adjustment to a chronic disabling illness in a family member. These include:

1. Is the family currently in crisis?
2. Has the family system changed to meet needs?
3. Is change acknowledged and accepted?
4. Who is assuming responsibility for what?
5. Is the assumed responsibility realistic?
6. Is the whole family involved in the plan?
7. Have family members' expectations been defined?
8. Is the current plan considered permanent or temporary?

The family described above would have greatly benefited from such an evaluation. The Smith family was in conflict, even with their dear mother, whom the older siblings were attempting to protect. The eldest son's frequent trips home to check on his mother resulted in Don neglecting his own family. His son's grades began to fall, and his four-year-old daughter was increasingly clinging and demanding; his wife wasn't too happy, either. The family system was attempting to change, with Don attempting to become the head of the family, but both Mrs. Smith and the youngest son were resisting change and ignoring the obvious declining ability of Mrs. Smith to manage her affairs. Don attempted to accept full responsibility for his mother, but this was unrealistic given that he lived several hundred miles away and had young children of his own that needed care. Although the middle daughters were supportive of Don, they had not recognized the need to share the responsibility. The family had not gotten together to discuss the issues and no formal plan was in place.

Problem-solving skills are essential in making successful adjustments and adaptations to a chronic illness such as Parkinson's disease. The problem-solving skills suggested by Zarit (Zarit, Orr, and Zarit, 1985) would be a helpful framework in dealing with the situation assessed for this family. The steps in the problem-solving process include:

1. Identifying the problem
   a. Antecedents
   b. Consequences
2. Generating alternative solutions (no censoring)
3. Selecting a solution and evaluating its pros and cons
4. Conducting a "cognitive rehearsal" of the plan
5. Carrying out the plan
6. Evaluating the outcome.

In the example provided above, the use of this problem-solving process eased the Smith family conflict. Don's wife insisted that something be done to reduce Don's excessive absences from home. Don called a family meeting and invited a counselor to help mediate. With the help of the counselor, the family was able to identify several problems. Don was away too much from home. Kenny's living at home resulted in extra work for his mother, although it did provide her company. Kenny did not feel capable to rent his own apartment and didn't have enough money to live in a nice place. The middle daughters did not like to go to their mother's to help out because they were too angry with Kenny and didn't really know how to help their mother. No long-term planning had been done. Although Mrs. Smith was no longer running the family business, there continued to be stressful expectations that she be involved in solving problems in the business. At the same time, Don felt responsible for managing problems in the business, although he had his own career and lived far away.

Once a list of problems had been identified, the family was invited to brainstorm possible solutions. All ideas were written down for consideration; no ideas were rejected or censored at this time. As the ideas were presented, the most possible and useful ones began to surface. Kenny still had difficulty with any suggestions that he do anything differently; he thought everything was fine the way it was. Mrs. Smith also tended to resist ideas that changed things from the way they had always been. After some discussion, the older siblings agreed that Don was doing too much and the other siblings were doing too little. The middle daughters were happy to accept more responsibility, if it was made clearer to them what they needed to do to help. The siblings and Mrs. Smith were able to agree that the business was too difficult for any of them to manage; with much sadness, they decided it was time to sell. Mrs. Smith was unwilling to sell her home and move in with any of her children, but she was willing to spend several months in the home of each of them. A proposed schedule of visitation was worked out. Kenny would still live in the family home, but when his mom was staying at home, a woman would be hired to cook and clean and assist Mrs. Smith with dressing and other activities. Mrs. Smith agreed to appoint Don to be in charge of her finances. The family recognized the benefit of joining a Parkinson support group to learn more about how to care for their mother as she became more disabled. Another meeting was scheduled in three months to review the progress of their plan.

When the family met three months later, the relationships between the siblings and with their mother were all improved. There was less tension, and an excitement and relief that everyone knew what to expect. Although the business had not been sold, Don had met with several possible buyers. A woman had been hired to come once a week to the house for cleaning, with the understanding that after the business was sold, full-time help might be needed. Mrs. Smith was invited to dinner at least once a week by the daughters, who also took over grocery-shopping for their mother. Kenny had not made many changes, but he did try to cook for his mother and seemed to be more aware of her limitations. Mrs. Smith was looking forward to spending the fall with her oldest son and his family. All of the problems had not been solved, but the family felt confident that they had found a way to identify and deal with problems as they arose and as Mrs. Smith's changing physical condition demanded new solutions.

THE IMPORTANCE OF SEEING THE FAMILY AS A UNIT

Medical personnel do not have an individual patient, but must treat and support a caregiver/care receiver unit, whether the unit is a husband and wife or parent and children. Effective education regarding disease process, prognosis, symptom management, and stress management for the Parkinson's patient and his or her caregiver(s) are critical for families managing disability and possible dementia in a loved one. Support and referral for specialized services can be provided to reduce the burden and alleviate the stress associated with caregiving. Respite services can be extremely helpful for many families. Similarly, professional recognition of depressive symptoms in both care receiver and caregiver is critical so that medication management and referral for mental health services can occur. A caregiver who is overwhelmed with stress may not be able to provide adequate care for his or her family member, which contributes to a downward spiral for both patient and family. Recognition of early signs of frustration and depression in a caregiver is an essential part of medical management.

THE INTERFACE OF THE FAMILY AND THE HEALTH CARE SYSTEM

A genuine systems perspective must recognize the reciprocal influences of the individual, the family, and other systems. The medical community is a primary system that families must negotiate when one of their members is diagnosed as having Parkinson's disease. It is critical that the health care professional dealing with these families address the impact of the illness and the stress of caregiving with preexisting or current stresses in designing clinical care for families. Family-oriented professionals must appreciate what it means for families to have a member develop serious and long-term disability, and how difficult it is for families to cope over time, especially when they shoulder the burden of primary caregiving. The medical community can respond to this need by seeing that appropriate mental health services are available. Services should include crisis intervention, brief, problem-focused family therapy, and multiple family groups. Additionally, mental health professionals dealing with the families of Parkinson's patients need specific information about the symptoms, progress, and treatment of the disease in order to provide the family with emotional support, information, and referral to needed resources such as support groups, home and respite care services, and nursing homes. The successful collaboration of physicians and mental health professionals can help parkinsonian patients and their families in achieving optimal adjustment.

SUGGESTED READINGS

Archbold, P. G., Stewart, B. J., Greenlick, M. R., and Harvath, T. (1990). "Mutuality and preparedness as predictors of caregiver role strain." *Research in Nursing and Health* 13:375–84.

Dakof, G. A., and Mendelson, G. A. (1986). "Parkinson's disease: The psychological aspects of a chronic illness." *Psychological Bulletin* 99:375–87.

Drinka, T. J. K., Smith, J. C. and Drinka, P. J. (1987). "Correlates of depression and burden for informal caregivers of patients in a geriatric referral clinic." *Journal of the American Geriatrics Society* 35: 522–25.

Grinspoon, L., ed. (1988). "Family therapy—Part I." *The Harvard Medical School Mental Health Letter* 4:1–4.

Karpel, M., and Strauss, E. (1983). "The family life cycle." In *Family Evaluation*. New York: Gardner Press, Inc, pp. 49–77.

Hainsworth, M. A., Eakes, G. G., and Burke, M. L. (1994) "Coping with chronic sorrow." *Issues in Mental Health Nursing* 15:59–66.

Lindgren, C. L. (1996). "Chronic sorrow in persons with Parkinson's and their spouses." *Scholarly Inquiry for Nursing Practice* 10:351–66.

Minuchin, S. (1977). *Families and Family Therapy*. Cambridge, Mass.: Harvard University Press.

Montalvo, B., and Thompson, R. (1988). "Conflicts in the caregiving family." *The Family Therapy Networker* (July/August): 30–35.

Strawbridge, W. J., and Wallhagen, M. I. (1991). "Impact of family conflict on adult child caregivers." *The Gerontological Society of America* 31:770–77.

Wallhagen, M. I., and Brod, M. (1997). "Perceived control and well-being in Parkinson's disease." *Western Journal of Nursing Research* 19:11–31.

Walsh, F., and Anderson, C. (1987). "Chronic disorders and families: An overview." *Journal of Psychotherapy and the Family* 3:3–32.

Zarit, H., Orr, N., and Zarit, J. (1985). *The Hidden Victims of Alzheimer's Disease: Families Under Stress.* New York: New York University Press.

4

Psychiatric Aspects

Terry McMahon

Since James Parkinson's original description of "the shaking palsy" in 1817, the disease that bears his name has long been recognized as a neurologic illness that can significantly and adversely affect the lives of patients and families. Some estimates suggest that as much as one percent of the U.S. population over age fifty may develop the core syndrome.

While neurological symptoms are widely recognized and associated with Parkinson's disease, psychiatric symptoms may be less commonly recognized. Historically, this phenomenon can be related to several factors. Parkinson himself initially excluded intellectual changes as a part of the syndrome. Likewise, subsequent reports often did not give particular attention to other psychiatric symptoms as a part of this disease.

However, reports over the last several decades have documented that a significant number of parkinsonian patients may manifest prominent psychiatric symptoms. This heightened recognition of psychiatric symptoms may relate to several factors: (1) a general increase in life expectancy, which may allow the disease to develop further and manifest these symptoms; (2) advances in drug therapies, i.e., dopaminergic and anticholinergic agents, which may, in addition to their therapeutic effects, produce significant psychiatric side effects; and (3) an increased awareness of how disease processes affecting the human nervous system may also foster changes in behavior, personality, and mood.

This chapter will attempt to describe the significant psychiatric symptoms that can be associated with Parkinson's disease and will include: (1) psychiatric symptoms prior to and during early phases of Parkinson's disease; (2) psychiatric symptoms associated with the middle and later phases of the disease; and (3) those symptoms that may be side effects of treatment. Finally, some comments regarding the management of these symptoms will conclude the discussion.

PSYCHIATRIC SYMPTOMS PRIOR TO AND DURING EARLY PHASES

While it is tempting to identify typical predisease personality changes in parkinsonian patients, a specific change in personality has yet to be identified. Earlier in this century, some writers entertained the notion that psychogenic and personality variables were primarily and causally related to the onset of Parkinson's disease. Such theories have now been widely abandoned. Nevertheless, in speaking with patients, clinicians have noted a tendency in some patients to be obsessive, reserved, self-critical, inflexible, and socially withdrawn. Such descriptive terms suggest possible psychological and behavioral features that correlate with the neurological picture, in which muscular rigidity and reduced movement often become prominent. However, these correlates, even if consistently present, have yet to be linked to neurological conditions associated with Parkinson's disease. Hence, for now, while investigators continue in their attempts to establish the consistency or specificity of these personality and behavioral attributes, we must remain cautious in attributing these changes to the underlying condition of the nervous system.

From a symptomatic standpoint, clinicians have also noted that depression and vague physical complaints (e.g., depressed mood, decreased self-esteem, tiredness, malaise, decreased energy, and minor aches and pains) may be prominent prior to and during early phases of the disease. Such symptoms are often nonspecific and, early on, may be attributed to poor diet, poor sleeping patterns, or arthritis. However, given these possible associations, the presence of such symptoms may warrant serious consideration of Parkinson's disease in patients who have no prior psychiatric history. This may be particularly important if relatives note any changes in gait, posture, or speech, as the patients themselves are often unaware of these subtle neurological changes early in the course of Parkinson's disease.

Finally, it should be noted that levels of awareness may be mildly affected in the early stages of the disorder. Difficulty in responding to shifting ideas while at the same time maintaining general mental acuity has been described in patients in early phases of the disease. These changes have also been linked to the "obsessive" personality features described above. Again, while specific, reliable findings have yet to be established, reports by families or patients of slowness in thinking, problem solving, or recall of memories—particularly when they coexist with vague physical or neurological symptoms, as noted above—may warrant consideration of Parkinson's disease.

PSYCHIATRIC SYMPTOMS ASSOCIATED WITH THE MIDDLE AND LATER PHASES OF THE DISEASE

The psychiatric syndromes that have been most commonly linked with this phase of Parkinson's disease include depression and dementia. However, in addition, anxiety, sleep disorders, and acute psychotic disorders have also been described.

Depression in particular has received increased attention because of research that has explored the neurological and chemical foundations of both depression and Parkinson's disease. Depression has been linked to changes in the central nervous system's ability to process norepinephrine and serotonin (two major kinds of neurotransmitters), while Parkinson's disease has been associated with diminution of dopamine levels in specific areas of the brain. Since the body processes dopamine and norepinephrine in a similar way, it has been tempting to link depression with Parkinson's disease at this neurochemical level. Moreover, dopamine depletion itself has been linked in animal models to behavior that would be viewed as a sign of depression if found in humans. Changes in serotonin metabolism have also been more recently linked with Parkinson's disease. However, until further research clarifies the significance of these findings, such relationships must remain hypothetical and speculative.

Estimates of the incidence of depression range as high as 90 percent, with most averages being in the area of 40 to 50 percent in parkinsonian patients. From a psychiatric perspective, certain aspects deserve specific comment. First, it can be useful to help patients and families differentiate problems with depressed mood, which may be more transient and reactive to the stress of the illness and its complications, from a true clinical depression in which the depressed mood is more sustained and accompanied by symptoms such as sleep disturbance (especially early morning awakening), appetite and weight changes, persistent negative or pessimistic ruminations about one's self or situation, lack of mood reactivity, and the presence of suicidal ideas. (These and similar symptoms are often referred to as *neurovegetative syndrome* because it affects the involuntary nervous system that controls body functions and glandular secretions.)

Second, given the overlap between the neurological symptoms of Parkinson's disease per se and neurovegetative symptoms commonly associated with depression, it may be especially important to focus on the nonphysical features of depression when considering a diagnosis of depression. More specifically, persistent negativism or pessimism, a negative view of self, lack of mood reactivity, and persistent early morning awakening may suggest that a superimposed depression exists that may deserve specific intervention.

Depression in particular has been an area of significant focus over the last decade in Parkinson's disease. Recent research has concluded the following. Biological factors intrinsic to the disease may be as much or more significant than psychological, reactive processes in the cause of depression. Parkinson's patients in particular may manifest much more sadness without guilt or self reproach. The relationship between depression and the severity of motor symptoms and physical disability may also be more limited than initially thought. Anxiety symptoms, including panic and phobic symptoms, may also coexist with depression and present clinically significant problems independent of depression. While earlier literature linked depression to later stages of illness, more recent data has suggested depressive signs and symptoms may also be a part of the picture in earlier stages of the disease. The association between laterality of motor symptoms and depression has also turned out to be confusing, with depression being associated with both left- and right-sided dominance in motor abnormalities. Finally, while depressive symptoms may occur at a relatively high frequency, many such patients will not meet diagnostic criteria for major depression and, hence, must be looked at more carefully in terms of decisions regarding antidepressant therapy.

Sleep disorders in Parkinson's disease have also been an area of increased interest in the last decade. Prevalence rates have ranged from 20 to 90 percent. A variety of problems have been reported, including problems with sleep onset, frequent awakenings, nightmares, daytime sedation, and fatigue. A variety of factors have been felt to be contributory, including the intrinsic motor disturbance, antiparkinsonian medications, anxiety and depression, and age, with older individuals sleeping less well. Optimal management of sleep problems is coming to be recognized as an important aspect of treatment. While antiparkinsonian medications have been associated with sleep problems, use of the same medications, which result in an improvement in motor symptoms, have also been associated with sleep improvement. Hence, interventions must be individualized to have an optimal affect for each patient.

Dementia has also been linked to the middle and later phases of Parkinson's disease. As noted by other contributors to this volume (e.g., see chapter 13), dementia may be defined as an acquired degeneration of general intellectual function related to brain dysfunction. A hypothetical distinction has been proposed between Alzheimer's disease as a so-called "cortical" dementia (localized on the surface or cortex of the brain) and Parkinson's disease as a so-called "subcortical" dementia (associated with an interior area of the brain). In addition to this differentiation based on location of the disease process in the brain, this hypothesis also suggests some differences in symptoms. Alzheimer's dementia may be characterized by aphasia (disorder of language due to brain dysfunction), amnesia (difficulty with recalling material), agnosia (failure to recognize or identify objects despite intact sensory function), apraxia (inability to carry out motor activities despite comprehension and motor function), and relative freedom from gait and motor dysfunction. In contrast, subcortical dementia may be characterized more by a relative lack of aphasia, more difficulty in retrieval of learned material (i.e., forgetfulness), slow problem solving, more personality and mood changes (i.e., depression and apathy), and prominent disturbances of gait and motor function.

While parkinsonian patients in the past were felt to be relatively free of dementia, a significant number of patients (some estimate as many as 20 to 80 percent) now are believed to develop symptoms of dementia. It may be especially useful to note that there appears to be a correlation between increased duration and severity of the Parkinson's disease and the severity of the symptoms of dementia.

Psychosis per se, as characterized by symptoms such as delusions, hallucinations, and mania, is relatively infrequent in Parkinson's disease. While up to one-fourth to one-third of patients may have visual hallucinations sometime during their illness, no specific association between Parkinson's disease and psychosis has been identified. Such symptoms have been more closely associated with insomnia and sleep disturbance, depression, delirium, dementia, and pharmacotherapy for Parkinson's disease (i.e., dopamine agonists). When hallucinations do occur, they are much more likely to be visual than auditory. Some patients may experience so-called benign hallucinations (also referred to as "Lilliputian" due to the hallucinations being of little people moving about the room) which are vivid, nonthreatening, and occur in the presence of intact insight and a clear sensorium. Appreciation of this is important in that such patients are not truly psychotic (i.e., they realize the hallucinations are not real and do not behave as if they were). Moreover, most antipsychotic medications are generally without benefit and their use may only serve to worsen the underlying motor symptoms of Parkinson's disease.

So-called paroxysmal disorders (sudden attacks of psychiatric symptoms) have also been attributed to the middle and later phases of the disease. These may include acute psychotic episodes with delusions and hallucinations that resemble either mania or schizophrenia, anxiety attacks, episodes (called perseverative episodes) involving a compulsion to perform tasks that involve the repeating of numbers or words, paranoia, and attacks of unusual or bizarre sensations in the extremities. In contrast to depression and dementia, such disturbances are felt to be less common and often abruptly resolve themselves after a short period of time without specific intervention.

PSYCHIATRIC SYMPTOMS RELATED TO DRUG THERAPY

Medications that enhance dopaminergic function (dopaminergic agents such as levodopa, bromocriptine, deprenyl, and amantadine) and medications that diminish cholinergic function (anticholinergic agents such as benztropine, trihexyphenidyl, and diphenhydramine) have been the mainstays of drug therapy in Parkinson's disease. Each of these major groups of medications have been linked to psychiatric symptoms.

Anticholinergic agents have the potential to produce a variety of psychiatric symptoms. Anticholinergic toxicity may manifest itself through such physical signs and symptoms as fever, hot and dry skin and mucous membranes, dry mouth, dilated pupils, distended abdomen, constipation, and retaining urine in the bladder. In addition, changes in psychiatric/mental status are often present and include confusion, disorientation, hallucinations (primarily visual), euphoria, and psychomotor agitation. It should be noted that elderly patients may be particularly susceptible to these medication side effects and may be further predisposed as a result of being prescribed several medications with anticholinergic properties. Patients with signs of dementia may also be predisposed to experience the adverse effects of these agents. It should be noted that many antidepressant and antipsychotic medications have these anticholinergic properties and can precipitate these symptoms when used in inappropriate dosages.

Dopamine toxicity can produce a characteristic syndrome including vivid dreams and nightmares, night terrors (characterized by thrashing and calling out during sleep and waking with prominent anxiety and fear without recall of the dream state), hallucinations (auditory and visual), delusions, paranoia, insomnia, elevated or hypomanic mood, and hypersexuality. A large number of the acute psychotic episodes experienced by parkinsonian patients may be linked to the effect of these dopaminergic medications. More than one-third of patients may develop some or all of these symptoms after two or more years of exposure to dopaminergic agents. Factors that may predispose patients to experiencing these side effects include dementia, older age, a history of prior episodes, increasing dosage of dopamine agonists, or use of larger numbers of medications which increase the likelihood of drug interactions. A progression of such symptoms has also been suggested, beginning with vivid dreams, nightmares, and night terrors, then progressing through hallucinatory experiences and paranoia. In particular it should be noted that the duration and severity of the parkinsonism may also be linked with a tendency toward these reactions and that patients with a prior history of schizophrenia may be susceptible to re-experiencing their psychotic symptoms as a result of exposure to these agents.

ASSESSMENT AND MANAGEMENT OF PSYCHIATRIC COMPLICATIONS

If parkinsonian patients develop any of the psychiatric symptoms noted above, a thorough and comprehensive evaluation is certainly warranted. Initially it is appropriate to take a history from the patient or family, which may particularly focus on whether there have been prior episodes or previous treatment for a major psychiatric disorder that could recur in the context of Parkinson's disease. If so, a history of effective treatment, both behavioral and cognitive as well as pharmacologic, should be elicited, since this will prove valuable in guiding future treatment.

If there is no history of prior psychiatric disturbance, it is important to rule out any physiological abnormalities that could produce these psychiatric symptoms. Many of the physiological changes that produce symptoms of delirium (confusion, disorientation, clouded consciousness) and dementia can also produce a variety of psychotic and psychological syndromes. If psychiatric symptoms are present, consideration should be given to a medical work-up similar to that for dementia or delirium. In addition, it should be kept in mind that a variety of nonparkinsonian medications can produce these psychiatric symptoms, including anti-anxiety agents (e.g., diazepam, chlordiazepoxide), antihypertensive agents, steroids, anti-ulcer agents (e.g., cimetidine), as well as antidepressant and antipsychotic medications. Hence, part of the evaluation of any psychiatric symptoms should be a careful review for other superimposed medical disorders and medications that may bring about the psychiatric symptoms noted.

If medication effects and/or interactions and other medical problems are ruled out, it is appropriate to consider several approaches to managing these symptoms. Nonpharmacologic interventions such as behavioral management, environmental restructuring, and supportive psychotherapy can be quite effective in this regard. Cognitive behavioral approaches and support groups can also be quite effective in helping to manage certain aspects of psychiatric symptomatology. The greater retention of language function relative to other areas (i.e., visuospatial) can be helpful in engaging patients in psychotherapy. In particular, the focus may be on issues such as self image, becoming more deliberate in planning movement and activities, and dealing with fears of humiliation. It is important to remind patients that they are often more "slow" than they are "impaired," and this may facilitate a more optimistic approach in adjusting to disabilities. However, if psychiatric symptoms are unresponsive to behavioral and/or other psychotherapeutic interventions, drug therapies are appropriate and should be prudently utilized.

In general, the choice of medications is related to the nature of the psychiatric symptoms as well as the status of the underlying Parkinson's disease. Initially, it may be most appropriate to consider a reduction of antiparkinsonian agents if possible. A reduction of anticholinergic medication may ameliorate symptoms of dementia or delirium, while reductions in dopaminergic medications may be effective for diminishing or extinguishing sleep disturbances, acute psychotic behavior with hallucinations and delusions, as well as associated paranoia. In general, if a patient has a prior history of schizophrenia, it may be preferable to use anticholinergic agents in treating the Parkinson's disease, since dopaminergic agents can likely exacerbate the underlying schizophrenia.

If the use of antipsychotic agents is deemed appropriate, medications such as chlorpromazine or thioridazine—both of which have more anticholinergic properties—may be less likely to exacerbate the Parkinson's disease. However, these same agents may be more likely to produce postural hypotension (a drop in blood pressure when rising to one's feet, which may produce dizziness and result in falls) and to produce signs and symptoms of anticholinergic toxicity and delirium. Dosages may need to be carefully measured and use limited to the shortest duration necessary to manage the symptoms. As noted above, antidepressant medication can also be usefully employed when depressive symptoms are more consistent and prominent in the clinical picture. Again, the more anticholinergic agents, such as imipramine or doxepin, may be better for Parkinson's disease, but they can produce side effects similar to antipsychotic medications. Antidepressants with lower anticholinergic potential (e.g., desipramine, maprotiline, and trazodone, which are also less sedating) may be more desirable.

Over the last decade, several new antipsychotics and antidepressants have been released and appear to be useful additions to the psychopharmacologic approaches to treatment. The so-called "atypical" antipsychotics (clozapine, risperidone, olanzapine) have been touted as useful agents due to their reduced side effects, including a reduced tendency to motor symptoms. Quetiapine, though currently less well studied, may also be a useful agent due to similar "atypical" properties. Although clozapine in particular has been linked to bone marrow suppression and therefore must be closely monitored, it has been shown to be effective in addressing signs and symptoms associated with psychosis and delirium. Some improvement in motor symptoms and disability has also been associated with its use. Among the newer antidepressants, specific serotonin reuptake inhibitors, the so-called SSRIs (i.e., fluoxetine, paroxetine, sertraline), and bupropion have also been used with positive results. These agents have also been touted for use due to their better side effect profiles. However, several cautions are noteworthy. SSRIs in particular may prolong the half-life of other medications. Hence, patients must be carefully monitored for drug interactions. In addition, some reports have noted worsening of parkinsonian symptoms with SSRIs. Bupropion, like the SSRIs, also tends to be a more stimulating agent and may enhance problems with agitation and sleep. Moreover, use of any antidepressant in association with deprenyl should be discouraged due to the potential for drug interactions. Finally, it should be noted that electroconvulsive therapy (ECT) continues to be a highly effective modality for treating depression and may be particularly beneficial when pharmacologic therapies are ineffective or contraindicated due to side effects. ECT has also been shown to have some positive impact in relieving motor symptoms, thus warranting further consideration of its use in certain instances.

While panic attacks are often responsive to treatment with antidepressants, benzodiazepines and anti-anxiety agents can also be useful for symptoms related to anxiety and sleep difficulties. If deemed appropriate, agents with shorter half-lives and no active metabolites (e.g., lorazepam, oxazepam, and alprazolam) are often preferable to benzodiazepines with longer half-lives and active metabolites (e.g., diazepam, chlordiazepoxide, clorazepate) in patients who are older. Buspirone is also a nonbenzodiazepine alternative for use as an anxiolytic. In general, the use of barbiturates (e.g., phenobarbital, secobarbital, amobarbital) should be avoided. They tend to produce paradoxical agitation, suppression of rapid eye movement (REM) sleep, and adverse drug interactions. Antihistamines (e.g., diphenhydramine) can be useful as sleeping agents but are also more likely to cause confusion and delirium and to exacerbate dementia because of their anticholinergic properties. Likewise, chloral hydrate can be useful as a sleeping agent, but it, too, has the potential for interacting with other medications that older patients may be taking (e.g., anticoagulants such as warfarin). Hence, adverse side effects and drug interactions should be borne in mind when considering drug therapies for anxiety or sleep problems.

CONCLUSION

In conclusion, psychiatric symptoms and disorders occur with sufficient frequency in parkinsonian patients to warrant familiarity with their manifestations and the factors that help to produce them. An awareness of how psychiatric problems present themselves and how each member of the health care team can contribute to more effective management of these problems will be useful to all who are involved in the treatment of patients with Parkinson's disease.

BIBLIOGRAPHY

Askenasy, J., and Yahr, N. (1985). "Reversal of sleep disturbance in Parkinson's disease by antiparkinsonian therapy: A preliminary study." *Neurology* 35:527–32.

Cummings, J., and Benson, D. F. (1984). "Subcortical dementia: Review of an emerging concept." *Archives of Neurology* 41:874–79.

Cummings, J. (1992). "Depression in Parkinson's disease: A review." *American Journal of Psychiatry* 149:443–53.

DeSmet, Y., et al. (1982). "Confusion, dementia, and anticholinergics in Parkinson's disease." *Journal of Neurology, Neurosurgery and Psychiatry* 48:1161–64.

Duvoisin, R. (1984). *Parkinson's Disease: A Guide for Patient and Family*, Second Edition. New York: Raven Press.

Factor, S., and Brown, D. (1992). "Clozapine prevents recurrence of psychosis in Parkinson's disease." *Movement Disorders* 7:125–31.

Fleminger, S. (1991). "Left-sided Parkinson's disease is associated with greater anxiety and depression." *Psychological Medicine* 21:629–38.

Fonda, D. (1985). "Parkinson's disease in the elderly: Psychiatric manifestations." *Geriatrics* 40:109–14.

Guze, B., and Bario, C. (1991). "The etiology of depression in Parkinson's disease patients." *Psychosomatics* 32:391–95.

Hantz, P., et al. (1994). "Depression in Parkinson's disease." *American Journal of Psychiatry* 151:1010–13.

Harvey, N. (1986). "Psychiatric disorders in parkinsonism." *Psychosomatics* 27:91–103 (Part 1) and 175–84 (Part 2).

Hauser, R., and Zesiewicz, T. (1997). "Sertraline for the treatment of depression in Parkinson's disease." *Movement Disorders* 12:756–59.

Inzelberg, R., Kipervasser, S., and Korczyn, A. (1998). "Auditory hallucinations in Parkinson's disease." *Journal of Neurology, Neurosurgery and Psychiatry* 64:533–35.

Koller, W., and Megaffin, B. (1994). "Parkinson's disease in parkinsonism." In *Textbook of Geriatric Neuropsychiatry*, C. Coffee and J. Cummings, eds. Washington, D.C.: American Psychiatric Press, pp. 433–56.

Klawans, H. (1978). "Levodopa-induced psychosis." *Psychiatric Annals* 8:447–451.

Kuzis, G., et al. (1997). "Cognitive functions in major depression and Parkinson's disease." *Archives of Neurology* 54:982–86.

Lees, A., and Smith, E. (1983). "Cognitive deficits in the early stages of Parkinson's disease." *Brain* 106:257–70.

Lieberman, A. (1998). "Managing neuropsychiatric symptoms of Parkinson's disease." *Neurology* 50 (Suppl. 6):S33–S38.

Maricle, R., et al. (1995). "Dose response relationship of levodopa with mood and anxiety in fluctuating Parkinson's disease: A double-blind, placebo-controlled study." *Neurology* 45:1757–60.

McNamara, M. (1991). "Psychological factors affecting neurological conditions." *Psychosomatics* 32:255–67.

Meco, G., et al. (1997). "Risperidone and levodopa-induced psychosis in advanced Parkinson's disease: An open label, long-term study." *Movement Disorders* 12:610–11.

Menza, N., and Rosen, R. (1995). "Sleep in Parkinson's disease: The role of anxiety and depression." *Psychosomatics* 36:263–66.

Naimark, D., et al. (1996). "Psychotic symptoms in Parkinson's disease patients with dementia." *Journal of the American Geriatrics Society* 44:296–99.

Richard, I., Kurlin, R., et al. (1997). "A survey of antidepressant drug use in Parkinson's disease." *Neurology* 49:1168–69.

Sanchez-Ramos, J., Ortoll, R., and Paulson, G. (1996). "Visual hallucinations associated with Parkinson's disease." *Archives of Neurology* 33:1265–68.

Schiffer, R., et al. (1998). "Evidence for atypical depression in Parkinson's disease." *American Journal of Psychiatry* 145:1020–22.

Siemers, E., et al. (1993). "Anxiety and motor performance in Parkinson's disease." *Movement Disorder* 8:501–506.

Smith, M., et al. (1997). "Sleep disturbances in Parkinson's disease patients and spouses." *Journal of the American Geriatrics Society* 45:194–99.

Stein, N., et al. (1990). "Anxiety disorders in patients with Parkinson's disease." *American Journal of Psychiatry* 147:217–20.

Tandberg, E., et al. (1997). "Risk factors for depression in Parkinson's disease." *Archives of Neurology* 54:625–30.

Tandberg, E., et al. (1996). "The occurrence of depression in Parkinson's disease." *Archives of Neurology* 53:175–79.

Thompson, T., Moran, M., and Nies, A. (1983). "Psychotropic drug use in the elderly." *New England Journal of Medicine* 308:134–38 (Part 1) and 194–199 (Part 2).

Trosch, R., et al. (1998). "Clozapine use in Parkinson's disease: Retrospective analysis of a large multi-centered clinical experience." *Movement Disorders* 13:377–82.

van Hilten, B., et al. (1994). "Sleep disruption in Parkinson's disease." *Archives of Neurology* 5:922–28.

van Hilten, J., et al. (1993). "Sleep, excessive daytime sleepiness and fatigue in Parkinson's disease." *Journal of Neural Transmission* 5:235–44.

Waters, C. "Managing the late complications of Parkinson's disease." *Neurology* 49 (suppl. 1):S49–S57.

Wirshing, W. (1995). "Neuropsychiatric aspects of movement disorders." In *Comprehensive Textbook of Psychiatry,* Sixth Edition, H. Kaplan and B. Sadock, eds. Baltimore: Willams and Wilkins, pp. 220–31.

Whitehouse, P., Freidland, R., and Straus, N. (1992). "Neuropsychiatric aspects of degenerative dementia associated with motor dysfunction." In *Textbook of Neuropsychiatry*, Second Edition, S. Yudofsky and R. Hales, eds. Washington, D.C.: American Psychiatric Press, pp. 593–97.

5

Parkinson's Disease and Its Impact on Sleep

Bhupesh H. Dihenia

It is well known that Parkinson's disease is related to the degeneration of some brainstem structures, particularly the substantia nigra and locus ceruleus. It is the degeneration of these structures with the depletion of dopamine that causes the manifestations of symptoms of Parkinson's disease, which include tremor, slowing of movements, rigidity, and postural instability. When there is significant dysfunction of these upper brainstem regions in producing neurotransmitters such as dopamine and norepinephrine, parkinsonian symptoms continue to worsen.

For many centuries, people thought that various diseases produced symptoms only during the waking period. With further understanding of sleep, however, we have discovered that most disorders have both waking and sleep components.

The generation of sleep and the control of wakefulness is related to the brainstem, especially the ascending reticular activating system. This is a region of diffuse brain cells along the brainstem that essentially acts as a switch to turn wakefulness on and off. Our knowledge of sleep disorders and even of normal sleep is still in its infancy. However, there have been numerous strides over the last twenty-five years which have allowed a greater understanding.

Sleep is divided into two main forms, non–rapid eye movement (NREM) and rapid eye movement (REM) stages. NREM sleep is subdivided into four stages. Stage I is a transition stage from wakefulness to sleep. Stage II is a little deeper, and stages III and IV are even deeper sleep. REM sleep is a separate state of sleep which is also considered part of deep sleep. It is believed that stages III and IV as well as REM sleep are restorative sleep.

In Parkinson's disease, there is degeneration of the brainstem structures. Sleep-control mechanisms are found in the brainstem, so it is not surprising that patients with Parkinson's disease have multiple sleep disorders. Although neurologists have a great understanding of the daytime waking symptoms of Parkinson's disease, there is still a significant neglect of treatment of the disease's nocturnal manifestations.

Some of the common sleep disorders associated with Parkinson's disease include:

- Insomnia—problems with sleep initiation (getting to sleep) and sleep maintenance (staying asleep).
- Disordered breathing—obstructive sleep apnea and/or upper airway resistance syndrome.
- Periodic limb movement disorder.
- REM behavior disorder.
- Restless leg syndrome.

The most common sleep disorder in the general population is insomnia. This is also a common sleep disorder associated with Parkinson's disease. Significant anxiety and panic disorders associated with Parkinson's disease may contribute to the insomnia. Significant rigidity and tremor may also cause some difficulty with sleep initiation and maintenance as well. Patients with Parkinson's disease may also have some concern about going to sleep and then waking up "frozen," unable to move or to take their morning doses of antiparkinson medications.

Patients with Parkinson's disease are at a high risk of having restless leg syndrome. This is a disorder in which an abnormal sensory disturbance in the legs exists that is temporarily relieved by movement of the legs. Frequent recurrences happen and are associated with almost constant periodic leg movements which can interrupt or prevent sleep. Many patients have such profound symptoms of restless leg syndrome that they pace the bedroom or the house in the hope of relieving the lower extremity sensory disturbance. Unfortunately, restless leg syndrome is relatively common among patients who have Parkinson's disease and can significantly impair their going to sleep.

Patients with Parkinson's disease are also highly susceptible to having affective mood disorders such as depression. Often patients with depression have significant difficulty with sleep initiation and maintenance. Other common symptoms of depression include loss of appetite, fatigue, and loss of interest in activities previously considered enjoyable.

Treatment of insomnia needs to be geared toward addressing the cause of the insomnia. If the cause is panic disorder or anxiety disorder, then pharmacological interventions can be helpful. If the cause of the insomnia is an affective mood disorder such as depression, antidepressants can be of significant benefit. If the insomnia is related to restless leg syndrome, then medications to address those symptoms can also alleviate the insomnia. If rigidity and tremor are the cause, then adequate nighttime treatment of the parkinsonian symptoms would help with the insomnia.

Often patients have insomnia related to a hyperarousal state. In these hyperarousal states, patients have a hard time "turning the mind off." In these situations the following suggestions might be helpful:

- Avoid daytime naps.
- Have a daytime physical activity and/or an exercise routine.
- Avoid stimulants such as coffee, tea, or other caffeinated beverages.
- Minimize fluid intake three to four hours prior to bedtime. This will help to limit the number of nighttime arousals from having to use the restroom.
- Write down plans for the following day. This allows one to plan and address the itinerary for the next day, relieving some of the anxiety.

Patients who have hyperarousal states that preclude sleep initiation also benefit from improved sleep hygiene. Sleep hygiene is a set of nocturnal or bedtime actions and behaviors that are optimal for sleep initiation and maintenance. Good sleep hygiene includes no activity in bed except for sleeping. One should not read, watch television, or eat in bed; bed should be associated with sleep and sleep only. Allow only 30 minutes to fall asleep; if the patient is still awake after 30 minutes, he or she should get out of bed and perform some monotonous activity such as reading, listening to music, etc. When the patient is finally sleepy, he or she should go to bed again. If the patient is unable to initiate sleep once again after 30 minutes, then he or she should get up again and repeat the monotonous activity. Another feature of good sleep hygiene is not having a clock in the bedroom that is visible from the bed. Often patients with insomnia will continue to watch the clock and become even more anxious that sleep has not come as time continues to pass. The bedroom should be kept dark and at a comfortable temperature to optimally help initiate sleep. Insomnia is a common problem, but with appropriate diligent planning it can be overcome.

Another common sleep disorder associated with Parkinson's disease is periodic limb movement disorder. This is very similar to the restless leg syndrome that occurs during the waking hours. Periodic limb movement disorder is a nocturnal disorder in which there is periodic rhythmic movements of the lower extremities (i.e., leg jerks) that often result in arousals. Obviously, the arousals are not necessarily that of being awake and conscious, but there is sleep state change and fragmentation of sleep which then can lead to daytime hypersomnolence (or sleepiness). These multiple arousals often do lead to significant daytime sleepiness. Treatments for restless leg syndrome or periodic limb movement disorder include the use of long-acting carbidopa/levodopa at bedtime, dopamine agonist, or clonazepam.

Another common sleep problem associated with Parkinson's disease is REM behavior disorder, a sleep disorder in which patients have a tendency to act out their dreams. There is significant motor activity during REM sleep. Some Parkinson's disease patients demonstrate REM behavior disorder prior to actually showing symptoms of Parkinson's disease itself. It is well known that this sleep disorder is often an early indicator of developing Parkinson's disease. Usually the patient's spouse will complain of the patient's bizarre behavior during the night. The patient has significant motor activity during sleep, such as thrashing the arms or legs so forcefully that they may even injure the spouse. In general, people dream during REM sleep; there is total paralysis of the body (except for the diaphragm) that precludes one from actually moving or acting out the dreams. In patients who have REM behavior disorder, the "switch" in the brainstem controlling movement is not turned off and motor activity occurs. Fortunately, with early diagnosis, treatment exists for this disorder which includes the use of long-acting carbidopa/levodopa or clonazepam at bedtime.

Patients with Parkinson's disease are also at risk of having sleep disordered breathing, in which there is some cessation of air flow during sleep. The lack of air flow leads to arousals. This disorder often leads to plummeting oxygen in the bloodstream as well. Sleep disordered breathing is a common disorder in the general population; unfortunately, due to the muscle rigidity experienced by patients with Parkinson's disease, they are at increased risk for this disorder. Treatment for sleep disordered breathing involves the use of a positive airway machine with a face mask that is worn at night. This machine keeps a certain amount of pressure in the airway and does not allow the airway to collapse. Other oral appliances for the treatment of sleep disordered breathing are in the early development stages.

Sleep disorders are common in patients with Parkinson's disease. The disturbance in both the normal amount and quality of sleep leads to chronic sleep deprivation. Sleep deprivation in turn leads to the worsening of daytime parkinsonian symptoms and also causes daytime hypersomnolence, irritability, and—rarely—cognitive impairment. These factors make the assessment and treatment of nocturnal difficulties in Parkinson's disease patients critical, indeed.

There are numerous treatments for sleep disorders in the Parkinson patient. Appropriate review by a physician of the clinical history is necessary, as is a physical examination and a review of medications. Often a polysomnogram (sleep study) is a valuable diagnostic tool. Much is known about sleep disorders, but unfortunately much more remains unknown. There is a need for further research and better understanding, as well as improved treatment of the sleep disorders already associated with Parkinson's disease. It is important to share sleep difficulties and symptoms with your neurologist. This will allow a better understanding of how the sleep disorders relate to Parkinson's disease so that appropriate treatment can be started to alleviate the problems and improve the quality of life. Hopefully, with a better understanding of the nocturnal events of sleep in Parkinson's patients, we will achieve a better understanding and treatment of Parkinson's disease overall.

6

Nursing Aspects of Parkinson's Disease
Janice Stewart and Angie Bednarz

Parkinson's disease is a progressive condition that requires a variety of strategies for managing its symptoms. The symptoms and problems of Parkinson's disease can vary from patient to patient and from day to day. One thing is certain: Nothing about Parkinson's disease ever stays the same. Fortunately, several effective medications are available to treat these symptoms, but it often becomes apparent that it takes more than just "pills" for successful control of disease symptoms—it takes an intense desire to take hold of the disease and fight back. The health care team and medications cannot alone manage Parkinson's disease and its symptoms. Self-help is essential. Money and time seem to be in shorter supply in today's world of HMOs and PPOs. As the face of medicine changes, so must the attitude of the consumer. It is time to be proactive, informed, and involved. This chapter presents many practical approaches to treatment and helpful hints in getting control of the troublesome symptoms of Parkinson's disease.

BE PREPARED:
A VISIT WITH THE DOCTOR

Typically, the Parkinson's disease patient will see a family physician, internist, or neurologist two to three times a year for ongoing care and management of the disease. Preparation for the visit is essential to get the most benefit from the often brief time that the patient has to cover a multitude of complaints and concerns or to obtain answers to the many questions that often arise as the illness progresses and changes through the years. The following is provided to assist the patient and family in establishing a mutually beneficial relationship with the physician and office staff. Hopefully, the end result will be improvement in quality of life through effective management of the illness.

Several weeks before the visit, begin to identify the primary concerns and problems that must be addressed. Make notes and write down a few specific questions. Are there bothersome side effects from the medications, motor fluctuations causing a decreased level of independence, or new symptoms present that are not understood? If possible, obtain additional information from a library, Parkinson's foundation, or local information center to study up on the disease. Research prior to the office visit can save both the physician and patient valuable time, and allows time to focus on other issues that might be more pressing. Knowledge is an essential tool in the fight against the ever-changing nature of Parkinson's disease!

Since Parkinson's disease symptoms can vary from time to time, it is often beneficial to bring a caregiver, a close family member, or a close friend to the office visit. Some symptoms that may not be noticed by the patient might be of great concern to a spouse or loved one. Depression, anxiety, and confusion are just a few problems that are sometimes denied or overlooked, when they may in fact be easily treated with the proper medications or medication adjustments.

Prepare a complete list of all medications that are currently being taken, including over-the-counter drugs and vitamins (even if these are not taken on a regular basis). List the name of each drug, as well as its strength and frequency taken; also note any drug-related allergies and a brief medical history, including major illnesses and surgeries. Be complete and update the list often. The physician will review the list of medications to minimize the chance of overdosing or drug-related interactions. It is also important to keep a copy of this list in an obvious place in the home, such as taped to the front of the refrigerator. Also, carry a duplicate list in the wallet or billfold in case of an emergency.

Management of Motor Fluctuations: Parkinson's Motor Diary

Three to five days before the visit begin monitoring motor function through the use of a Parkinson's Motor Diary (see next page). The motor diary is one method of assessing motor function, especially in those

PARKINSON'S DISEASE MOTOR DIARY

Complete the Motor Diary below for 3 to 5 days before your next doctor's visit

1. Place a check under each 30 minute time period to indicate if you are "ASLEEP," "ON," "OFF," or experiencing "DYSKINESIAS." Only one of these categories will be marked for each 30 minute period.
2. Check the time periods when you eat meals.
3. Indicate times when Parkinson's (P.D.) medications are taken. (List your P.D. meds. in the table below, then indicate the medication taken by placing the corresponding number under the time taken.)

TABLETS TAKEN: (Parkinson's medications only)

1 = _____   3 = _____
2 = _____   4 = _____

DATE	A.M.																P.M.																A.M.							
	5	30	6	30	7	30	8	30	9	30	10	30	11	30	12	30	1	30	2	30	3	30	4	30	5	30	6	30	7	30	8	30	9	30	10	30	11	30	12	30	1	30	2	30	3	30	4	30
Asleep																																								
On																																								
Off																																								
Dyskinesia																																								
Mealtime																																								
Tablets Taken																																								

Sometimes it's hard to choose just one level of functioning. Please keep the following in mind.

ASLEEP: If you are asleep, check this box only.
ON: P.D. meds. are working/P.D. symptoms decreased
OFF: P.D. meds. have worn off/P.D. symptoms increased
DYSKINESIAS: Fidgety, restless, involuntary body movements (NOT TREMOR!)

NAME/CHART # _____   DATE _____

Parkinson's disease patients who experience frequent and bothersome motor fluctuations. The patient is asked to record the level of motor function every 30 minutes during a 24-hour period by recording sleep time, "on" time (with or without dyskinesias), *or* "off" time. Meals and times of medication dosing are also noted on the diary by placing a mark under the approximate time that meals are eaten and Parkinson's medications are taken. The physician can review the diaries to determine if a pattern evolves in the patient's motor performance and analyze this performance in relation to medication. The physician can then adjust the dosage or timing of the medication accordingly.

On, Off, and In Between

Prior to completing the motor diaries, it is essential that both the doctor and patient are using the same terms to describe motor performance. The terms "on," "off," and "dyskinesias" are sometimes confusing, even for patients who have had Parkinson's disease a number of years.

"On" time is used to describe the period when the patient's Parkinson's disease medications are working. Movements are normal or almost normal, and the patient is in a relative state of good motor function. "On" time may also be associated with *dyskinesias.* Dyskinesias are abnormal, involuntary movements of the voluntary muscles, for example, in the arm, leg, or hand. Dyskinesias can vary greatly in pattern, from barely discernible twitches and jerks to twisting, writhing movements involving most of the body. Dyskinesias are frequently the result of too much levodopa in the body rather than too little. It is important not to confuse dyskinesias with tremor, for they are two different phenomena. Patients may be "on" and still have dyskinesias. If this is the case, only dyskinesias would be noted on the motor function diary for that time period.

Tremor is a rhythmic to-and-fro motion involving the arm, leg, jaw, lower facial muscles, or even the lips. This common symptom of Parkinson's disease occurs when the muscles are at rest and is commonly described as a "pill-rolling" motion involving thumb and finger movements. Tremor usually disappears during sleep and increases under stress. Tremor can occur without relationship to the Parkinson's disease patient's overall level of motor function. A person can be "on" or "off" and still have tremor, making it unreliable for determining motor fluctuation patterns. "On" is when the medication is working, not necessarily an absence of tremor.

When a person with Parkinson's disease starts treatment with levodopa/carbidopa, the effects are typically dramatic. The parkinsonian notices a great reduction in slowness, stiffness, and/or tremor, possibly to the extent that symptoms seem nonexistent. This "levodopa honeymoon" period usually lasts from two to five years. During this time, the patient usually does not feel any wearing off (reduction in benefits) of the medication. Eventually, however, many patients begin to experience a decrease in mobility or an increase in the tremor between doses. The level of motor function begins to fluctuate. This is known as the "wearing-off phenomenon." "Off" time is the period of time when medications are not working.

Wearing off may occur subtly: for example, when a person awakens in the morning and finds that the symptoms of the disease are particularly prominent. Wearing off can also occur routinely at the end of each levodopa dosing period. These are both examples of predictable end-of-dose motor fluctuations. More abrupt, rapid swings of "on/off" syndrome are unpredictable in nature and can occur at any time without relationship to when the Parkinson's medications are taken. Unfortunately, these unpredictable "off" periods are much more difficult to manage with medication adjustments alone. *Freezing* is an example of an abrupt "off" period that may range in severity from a brief hesitation of the feet to severe immobility.

Freezing is the name given to the temporary, involuntary inability to move and is fairly common among persons with Parkinson's disease. Some patients refer to freezing episodes as a "lock down." Freezing may occur at any time. When it happens, it seems one's feet "stick" to the floor or one is unable to get up from a chair. There are certain situations where a freezing episode might be likely to occur. Examples of situations include walking through doorways, getting on and off elevators, walking in crowds, or going up and down stairs. Freezing requires behavioral retraining to initiate movement and break the freeze. One way to move smoothly through the environment is to develop a "motor program." A motor program is an anticipated strategy for movement through areas that cause problems. If correctly anticipated, the attention required for the movement is lessened, and the stress and anxiety are reduced. As a patient continues to anticipate movement strategies, a preprogrammed approach is established for the next encounter with the same movements. Then all that is needed are small adjustments for new obstacles. For example, if the patient is going to walk down a hallway and through the bedroom door, the required movements are anticipated and performed the same way each time. However, if one's spouse is also coming up the hallway and the dog is at the bedroom door, some adjustments must be made. These obstacles can be anticipated and attention paid to them. Often, avoiding situations that cause freezing episodes may be the best defense. If in a frozen state, some suggestions to get out of it include:

- Stop trying to continue the activity.
- Call for help.
- Change direction. If unable to move forward, move sideways or take a step backward.
- Use a sound or rhythm to stimulate movement.
- Think of or sing a tune and then move to the beat. Marches have a good rhythm.
- Count silently or out loud and then move to the count: 1-2-3, 1-2-3.
- Visualize an object, then lift a foot and try to step over the imaginary object.
- Imagine floor tiles are stepping stones and try to step from one to the other.
- Use a pocket flashlight to throw a pool of light in front of the feet; try stepping into the pool.
- If a cane is used, draw an imaginary line on the floor and try stepping over the line.
- Ask a companion to place a handkerchief or piece of paper on the floor; try to step over the object.
- If there is a tendency to freeze in a specific place such as a doorway, try to visualize beyond the obstacle. Once beyond the object, freezing will not likely occur.

Mobility

Mobility, the ability to move in the environment, can pose many challenges to the parkinsonian, not only because of the disease symptoms but also because of changes associated with the aging process. Walking or getting in and out of a bed or a chair can be quite a chore. The following techniques can be utilized to make a variety of transfers easier and safer for the patient:

- *To transfer into a bed, a chair, or a car,* approach the seat as closely as possible, turn so that one's back is to the chair, bed, or car seat, and back up until the edge of the seat is felt against the back of the legs. To sit down, bend forward slightly and lower the body down to a sitting position. In a chair, use the arms of the chair for guidance and balance. To finish getting into a car, swing each leg into the car. Slide over in the seat to a comfortable position. A plastic bag or satin seat cover placed on the seat will make sliding easier, and a handle may be attached to the dashboard or door frame by an auto body shop to make the transfer easier. To complete getting into a bed, lift one leg at a time into the bed. Lie down slowly using arms for support (or lower the head of an electric bed). To move to the center of the bed, move the hips and then the shoulders until a comfortable position is achieved.

- *To transfer out of a chair,* place both feet slightly apart with the stronger foot in front of the other. Both feet will be partially under the front of the chair. Slide forward until positioned at the edge of the chair. Using the armrests, bend forward so that the nose is over the knees and push up while leaning forward. Straighten up slowly. Rocking back and forth several times may provide a slight boost to make this transfer easier.

- *To transfer out of a car,* slide to the outside edge of the seat, swing both legs out of the car, and place feet slightly apart on the ground. Lean forward and stand as if rising from a chair. Use the car door and frame for support, if necessary. Also, be sure the car is parked far enough from the curb so that one can step onto level ground before getting into or out of a car.

- *To transfer out of a bed,* turn onto one's side and scoot to the edge of the bed, alternately moving the hips and the shoulders a little at a time. Slide the feet off the edge of the bed and use the arms to push up into a sitting position. Once in the sitting position, assess whether any dizziness is experienced before continuing. A side rail may be helpful when getting out of a bed. With feet on the ground and partially under the edge of the bed, lean forward and push up to a standing position. It is wise to place a walker or sturdy piece of furniture at bedside for additional security during the transfer, if needed. Remember to place the stronger of the feet slightly in front of the other and to rock back and forth several times to help boost up more easily.

When *choosing a chair* to sit in, choose straight-back chairs with arms for easier movement into and out of them. Chair height should also be considered when choosing a good sitting chair, and *never* transfer into any chair with rollers or wheels unless precautions have been taken. If a chair has rollers, make sure someone is holding it steady to prevent an accident. During transfers to and from a wheelchair, always make sure the brakes are locked to prevent unanticipated movement of the chair during the transfer. Also remember that the more stuffing in the chair, the more difficulty one may have getting out of it. Electric tilt chairs can be a wise investment and often are covered by insurance.

If *bed transfers* are a problem, there are ways to make this task less difficult for the Parkinson's disease patient. Transfers can be made easier simply by adjusting the bed's height, either by raising it with blocks under the legs or lowering it by cutting the legs shorter. An electric bed can be very useful when transfers become increasingly more difficult, and insurance may cover part or all of this expense. Two assistive devices that are available include a trapeze bar that is suspended above the bed, and a grab bar secured to the wall beside the bed. Each of these devices can be found at a medical supply store and may also be covered by insurance. Satin or nylon sheets and pajamas make movement in bed much easier.

When *walking,* especially in an unfamiliar environment, assistive devices may be used for better mobility and stability. The use of a walking cane or hiking stick may lend support and aid in balance. The height of such a stick encourages the user to stand straighter and maintain a center of gravity. A cane may be difficult to use for a person with Parkinson's disease. The low height of the cane encourages leaning forward, which is very dangerous for people whose stooped posture already tends to cause the center of gravity to be shifted forward. The most secure device to use for gait problems is the walker. A walker with locking wheels that engage when weight is applied to the walker is recommended for ease in use and safety. A basket or bag can be attached to the front of the walker and used for carrying items such as a cordless telephone and medications. Other types of walkers are lightweight, aluminum-frame walkers with or without wheels. These walkers may not be as helpful if the user tends to fall backward. This walker also does not provide support for balance as the other walker does. For persons who are unsure of their balance or have had numerous falls, a wheelchair or electric scooter is recommended. These are especially useful when out in public and away from the home environment.

Dizziness: Orthostatic Hypotension

Many patients with Parkinson's disease experience a drop in blood pressure when changing from a lying or sitting position to a standing position. The medical term for this is *orthostatic hypotension.* Common symptoms include lightheadedness or dizziness, with or without feeling faint. Weakness and loss of consciousness can occur if the drop in blood pressure is severe. Orthostasis may be caused by medication side effects or may be a combination of aging and other existing diseases. The Parkinson's disease patient should consult with the physician if these symptoms occur. If dizziness or lightheadedness results with a change in positions, the following suggestions may be helpful:

- Sit on the edge of the bed or chair for a few minutes before getting up.
- Exercise feet and legs prior to rising from the bed or a chair.
- Stand up slowly, holding a sturdy piece of furniture or a walker.
- Keep the head of the bed tilted upward at a 30-degree angle.
- Consult with a physician about adding salt to food to help maintain blood volume.
- Drink a cup of regular coffee after meals.
- Eat small, frequent meals (4-6 per day).
- Sit down after exercise to prevent pooling of blood in the feet.
- Wear elasticized stockings (thigh high are recommended) to promote blood return from the feet and legs back to the heart.

If these measures fail and the problem becomes severe, the physician may prescribe medication to maintain adequate blood pressure. Report all symptoms to a physician for available treatment options.

Recovery from a Fall

Falling is a very real consequence when Parkinson's disease affects gait and balance. People at risk for falling should practice recovery from a fall. It is helpful to have someone on hand when practicing in case there is difficulty getting up, even from the practice session. To begin, the patient should lie on the floor as if a fall occurred, and follow these steps:

- Remain still for a few moments to calm the nerves.
- Move the arms and legs slowly to see if there is any injury. If there is extreme pain, be careful not to further injure the site.
- Turn to a sidelying position and place the hands on the floor with palms down. By "walking" the hands up to the waist, one can get to a sitting position.
- Sit in this position for a moment while checking again for injury.
- Turn over onto the hands and knees and crawl to a sturdy chair.
- Position a hand on either side of the chair seat.
- Bend the strongest leg at the knee, placing the foot flat on the floor.
- Push up to a standing position.
- Turn around slowly and sit on the chair.

If a fall occurs and the patient is unable to get up and sit on the chair, attempt to crawl to a telephone and call for assistance. If the patient is unable to crawl, attempt to move across the floor by scooting on one's back or side to a telephone.

Exercise

Exercise is critical for Parkinson's disease patients to achieve the most independent and active lifestyle possible. Do not give up the activities of enjoyment: walk, play sports, shop, play cards, garden, cook. Each of these activities has a level of exercise to it and contributes to physical and mental well-being. The key for exercise is to establish a program that is enjoyable, start at a slow pace, and build up to a comfortable level. The more enjoyable an exercise program, the longer a person will continue to exercise. Make the exercise a social event. A partner or a group will enhance commitment to the activity. A pet can make a wonderful companion when walking.

To reduce rigidity and stiffness, stretching exercises are recommended on a daily basis. Stretching promotes flexibility. Yoga and Tai Chi are beneficial stretching exercises. Strengthening exercises work on the large muscles of the body (arms, legs, abdomen, etc.) to keep the body in tone. These exercises generally involve the use of light weights. The Parkinson's disease patient should seek the advice of a physical therapist or exercise trainer for these activities. At some institutions, there are programs with physical therapy and occupational therapy designed with Parkinson's disease needs in mind. Aerobic activity includes exercises such as walking, running, swimming, cycling, and others. Since aerobic activity does put stress on the body, please consult with a physician before starting the program. If exercising at home, remember to stretch before and after each session.

Nutrition

Parkinson patients often have concerns about daily nutrition. In general, the parkinsonian patient should attempt to maintain a well-balanced diet with a daily menu based on whole grains, fruits and vegetables, calcium-rich foods, and protein foods. However, the parkinsonian patient should be aware that there are some changes that may need to be made to maintain overall health and maximal functioning in activities of daily living.

Gastric motility decreases with Parkinson's disease and constipation is a very common complaint. Swallowing is prolonged and the stomach may take longer to empty than before. For these reasons, it is often beneficial to consume small meals frequently throughout the day rather than three large meals. Increased fiber intake by eating foods such as bran, leafy vegetables, and fruits may be beneficial to combat constipation. Prune juice may also aid constipation.

An adequate fluid intake is necessary for preventing constipation, urinary tract infections, and kidney infections. As one ages, the natural sense of thirst diminishes; therefore, the Parkinson's disease patient must be sure to drink the required amount. The risk of dehydration is lowered with adequate intake of fluids, and it also enhances the absorption of nutrients and medications. Eight glasses of fluid a day are required for proper body function. A tip for keeping up with fluid intake is to schedule fluid intake as you schedule medication intake. For example, drink one eight-ounce glass of water every hour from 7 A.M. until 2 P.M. This will assure that the fluid requirement is met and that it is met early enough in the day to avoid getting up for the bathroom frequently during the night. Any fluid after 2 P.M. will be extra benefit.

In general, a multiple vitamin with mineral supplement is a good addition for general nutrition benefits. Other vitamins and minerals to include daily are calcium, vitamin D, and magnesium. Getting calcium and vitamin D can be difficult since milk and cheese also have high amounts of protein and may alter levodopa absorption. Eating cereal and orange juice fortified with calcium and magnesium will assist in receiving the needed 1,200 to 1,500 mg. of calcium a day. Calcium supplements also are beneficial. Calcium carbonate is often not tolerated well; however, calcium citrate is well tolerated, though chewable tablets are better absorbed. Vitamin D is essential for calcium absorption and can be found in enriched cereals and milk. One also produces Vitamin D when exposed to sunshine. Magnesium helps rebuild and strengthen bone and acts as a natural muscle relaxant. Magnesium is found in dark green vegetables, beans, peas, and whole grains.

Weight loss is common among Parkinson's disease patients and can lead to risks for illness, bone fractures, and general muscular weakness. Tremor, dyskinesias, difficulty swallowing, and bradykinesia may all contribute to decreased nutritional intake because eating becomes very difficult with these symptoms. Other factors contributing to weight loss are the medication side effects of nausea and loss of appetite. Furthermore, general fatigue and depression can play a role in weight loss. Muscle rigidity and tremor increase the calories utilized by the body and further add to weight loss. Frequent small meals and snacks may help maintain weight. Schedule plenty of time for meals to be eaten. Choose soft foods such as meatloaf, stew, and cooked vegetables for times when stiffness, slowness, and tremor are bothersome. It can be very discouraging if the Parkinson's disease symptoms are present and one is attempting to eat steak and a salad. Keep enjoyable foods available. If the

Parkinson's disease patient is eating a balanced diet and still loses weight, caloric intake may need to be increased. A liquid food supplement is a good way to add additional calories to one's daily intake. A Parkinson's disease patient should drink three to four cans of supplement a day as well as eat three well-balanced meals to meet requirements for weight gain or weight maintenance. A supplement can also add to daily nutritional requirements with the addition of fruit. Add chopped ice and fruit to a vanilla supplement and blend to make a smoothie. For a morning treat, add chopped ice, instant coffee, and chocolate syrup to a chocolate-flavored supplement and blend.

If nausea resulting from medications is a problem, take medications with a small snack such as crackers or pretzels. The addition of carbidopa (Lodosyn) prescribed from the physician may also relieve the nausea that may accompany intake of levodopa. Generalized nausea not related to medication intake will require a consultation with an internist or gastrointestinal physician to eliminate other possible causes. Swallowing difficulties for Parkinson's disease patients may also complicate matters. Consult a speech pathologist for a swallowing evaluation. The speech pathologist should be able to offer helpful advice to make swallowing easier and avoid choking episodes. If one has difficulties with being overweight, a reduction in calories may be required. If you have difficulties with weight loss or weight gain, report this to your physician, who may make a referral to a nutritionist.

Protein may interfere in the absorption of Parkinson's disease medications for a small percentage of people. Protein can block the absorption of levodopa, causing the feeling that "the medication is just not kicking in." If this is a problem, a redistribution of protein intake during the day may be required. To redistribute daily protein, one does not need to decrease the amount of protein in the diet. Patients have found that eating small amounts of protein in the morning and afternoon and leaving the remainder of daily protein for dinner is beneficial. Parkinson's disease symptoms may be more pronounced in the evening because the levodopa may not be absorbed as well. Patients find that they can set a routine of relaxation (reading a book, watching television) until bedtime and adjust to the protein redistribution well. The high-protein foods to be redistributed during the day include milk, red meat, fish, poultry, cheese, eggs, nuts, whole grains, some cereal, and soybean products. Another diet strategy for protein redistribution is a ratio of carbohydrates to protein taken at each meal. For example, a 7:1 ratio means 7 parts carbohydrates and 1 part protein at a meal. This may allow for a more regular meal than leaving all protein for the evening meal. One would have a small amount of meat, poultry, fish, milk, cheese, or eggs and a large amount of fruits, grains, and vegetables at each meal. A registered dietitian can help with a diet that is right for each individual Parkinson's disease patient.

Constipation

Constipation is a common complaint among people with Parkinson's disease. There are several reasons for this uncomfortable problem. Parkinson medications can worsen constipation and the muscles of the bowel slow down from the disease. In addition, parkinsonians tend to exercise less frequently as their muscles become tight and stiff. Finally, Parkinson's disease patients tend to drink insufficient amounts of fluids and include too little fiber in their diet.

To determine if constipation is a real problem, it is important to understand the terms that are frequently associated with this condition. First, "normal" bowel function is defined as having regular bowel movements. A schedule of "regular" bowel movements for one person may be one every three days, but for another person it may be one every day. The Parkinson's disease patient must consider what has been "regular" in the past and then determine if a problem now exists. Constipation is not only a change in the frequency of bowel movements but also in the consistency (hard, dry, difficult-to-pass stools). Fecal impaction is the occurrence of hard, dry stool accumulated in the colon and not passed. The following are several safe and simple steps for the prevention and treatment of constipation:

- *Eat high-fiber foods:* Whole grain cereals and breads, bran, whole raw fruits, and leafy vegetables are high-fiber foods that should be included in the diet. There are a variety of bran products available that can be added to fruit or breakfast cereal daily. The addition of a high-fiber liquid food supplement will not only increase fiber, but also add valuable calories if weight loss is a concern. Fiber can stimulate bowel function, because it acts like a sponge and draws water into the intestine to make the stool larger, softer, and easier to pass. There should be a gradual increase of fiber in the diet to avoid abdominal discomfort.
- Use natural constipation relief. One effective method is a prune juice cocktail, which can be made with 2 cups applesauce, 2 cups bran, and 1 cup prune juice. Mix together and store in refrigerator. Take 1 tablespoon every morning and gradually increase each morning until an effective dose is found.

- *Drink 8 to 10 glasses of water a day.* Water, like fiber, helps to keep the stools softer. Coffee, tea, cola, and alcohol dehydrate the body and are therefore not good substitutes for water. By putting a pitcher of water into the refrigerator every morning and emptying it by the end of the day, the daily fluid requirement is fulfilled. To prevent having to get up during the night, it is helpful if fluid intake is limited after midafternoon.
- *Exercise.* Exercise stimulates bowel function, so an increase in the daily activity level will be beneficial in the treatment and prevention of constipation. Consult with a physician to establish a regular exercise program.
- *Establish a time* each day for regular bowel movements (or every two or three days, if this is a regular schedule).
- *Do not ignore* or put off the urge to go.
- *Use bulk-forming laxative.* These are effective, but one must remember to take in the fluid requirement every day. Bulk formers may cause gas or increased constipation. Metamucil and Perdiem may be purchased without a prescription.
- *Use stool softeners.* The water content of stool is increased with these medications to produce larger and softer stools that are easier to pass. Colace, Doxidan, and Surfak are examples of stool softeners that may be purchased without a prescription.
- *Use stimulant laxatives.* Laxatives are most effective when used under the advice of a physician. The Parkinson's disease patient should try the more natural dietary strategies before taking laxatives. Follow directions carefully, for some laxatives can be harmful to the bowel and can damage the lining of the colon over time. Milk of Magnesia, Lactulose, and magnesium citrate are examples of stimulant laxatives.

In addition to stimulant laxatives, constipation may be treated by using glycerin suppositories and enemas. These remedies must be closely monitored by a physician, and should only be used as a last resort.

Restoration of normal bowel function usually takes two to three months. Constipation can be overcome by patiently establishing a consistent routine and maintaining the routine once successful relief of constipation is reached.

Voiding Difficulties

Some Parkinson's disease patients are faced with urinary discomforts and difficulties such as nocturia (having to void during the nighttime), frequency and urgency to urinate, and feeling of incomplete emptying of the bladder. Retention of urine leading to urinary tract infections, bladder spasms, and enlarged prostates for men are each problems that may require a visit with a urologist; however, all symptoms may benefit from consultation with a physician. In addition, it is suggested that fluid intake be decreased in the late afternoon and evening hours to aid in decreasing the trips to the bathroom during the night. A bedside commode or urinal may also be useful for voiding at night. In the event of incontinence (bed-wetting), adult diapers may be used or, for men, a condom catheter can be placed for the night. Drinking a glass of cranberry juice daily may assist in the prevention and treatment of urinary tract infections. Parkinson's disease medications may contribute to voiding difficulties. A discoloration of urine is noted with medications such as tolcapone. This is not a harmful side effect of the drug; however, the patient should report any changes in urinary status to the physician.

Changes in Mood and Mental Status

When living with Parkinson's disease, patients often are faced with dealing with symptoms of depression and anxiety. These are two areas that may easily be controlled, but one must report such symptoms to the physician.

Depression is a normal consequence of facing life with a chronic, debilitating disease. Parkinson's disease patients are frustrated by muscular rigidity, slow movements (bradykinesia), and shaking (tremor) that interfere with one's ability to perform activities. Antidepressants are frequently prescribed for treatment of depression in Parkinson's disease. Antidepressants may also relieve some of the symptoms of Parkinson's disease when initiated. Many patients also notice a lessening of depression with the initiation of levodopa treatment; however, further treatment with antidepressants may be necessary. There are also many interventions to fight depression, such as physical activity. Patients should remain as active as possible and avoid isolation. Some suggestions include exercise, crafts, gardening, volunteer work, church activities, and support group meetings. Identify goals (start small) and strive to accomplish them. Increase individual expectations and goals slowly and keep them realistic and specific in nature so that the goals may be accomplished. Set a time frame for completion of each goal and evaluate the progress.

Anxiety can also have an impact on an individual's Parkinson's disease symptoms. A key to dealing with anxiety is being able to recognize the part that stress plays in one's life and being willing to make the changes necessary to reduce stress and anxiety. Planning the day's activities can help reduce anxiety by giving one control over tasks to accomplish and events to attend. Avoid deadlines if possible, because they can be particularly distressing. Allow plenty of extra time for scheduled activities or outings. Get plenty of sleep. After a very busy day, it is helpful to schedule a day of rest to recuperate. For some patients, eating and drinking alcohol in moderation, monitoring caffeine intake, and discontinuing smoking may relieve some anxiety. By putting items in the same place every day, one may avoid last-minute panic when trying to locate keys or a wallet.

Although everything is done to avoid anxiety, it often occurs anyway. A few approaches to cope with anxiousness include deep breathing, progressive relaxation, and biofeedback. Keeping a daily journal provides a way to unburden oneself and to keep track of daily functioning. Relaxation tapes and books discussing relaxation methods are available in bookstores and libraries.

When faced with either depression or anxiety, maintain open communication with your nurses and physician. In addition, strive to improve communication with family members by discussing feelings of fear, loneliness, embarrassment, and frustration. Counseling with a psychologist or psychiatrist may also be of benefit for the Parkinson's disease patient struggling with depression and/or anxiety.

A Parkinson's disease patient may develop some changes in his/her overall mental status. This change may be in the form of confusion, visual hallucinations, or agitation as observed by the caregiver or family members. Parkinson's disease medications or some combination of other medications could be contributing to these behavioral changes, and it is best to contact the physician for advice.

For further information on these aspects, please refer to chapter 2, "Emotional Changes in Parkinson's Disease," and chapter 4, "Psychiatric Aspects."

Small Handwriting

Many Parkinson's disease patients notice difficulty with handwriting as an initial symptom. This symptom relates to the rigidity (stiffness) and bradykinesia (slowness) in the hands that goes along with Parkinson's disease. Small handwriting, or micographia, may improve with the onset of levodopa therapy. If handwriting is still bothersome, it is often beneficial to exercise the hands with small muscle exercises such as squeezing a soft ball in the palm of the hand, putting silverware away, or picking up pennies from a table. Sewing or crocheting are also ways for exercising the hands. Try different types of pens, thicker versus thinner, felt-tip versus ballpoint, to determine which pen is easier to use. Another hint to combat small handwriting is to use wide lined paper when corresponding. If handwriting starts to get smaller as it progresses, pick up the hand and start again. If one is unable to write, a tape-recorded message or a type-written letter would be alternative methods to stay in contact with family and friends. If all else fails, make a telephone call.

Drooling and Dry Mouth

The buildup of saliva is a common occurrence for Parkinson's disease patients. The swallowing reflex is normally automatic; however, this autonomic reflex is reduced in Parkinson's disease and saliva tends to build up in the mouth and throat. If this occurs, the saliva may spill out between the lips and drooling results. Although the Parkinson's disease patient assumes there is an overproduction of saliva, the problem is actually the failure to swallow at a normal rate. To combat this problem, it is helpful to make a conscious effort to swallow often, and to attempt to keep the head in an upright position (good posture) so the saliva will collect in the back of the throat and possibly stimulate a swallow. Chewing sugarless gum and sucking on hard candy may also stimulate a swallow.

Some patients with Parkinson's disease experience dry mouth due to reduced or thickened saliva. The most common cause of dry mouth is as a side effect of medication (usually anticholinergics). Other factors contributing to dry mouth are difficulty swallowing and keeping the mouth open while awake or asleep. Dry mouth can lead to gum disease and cavities, so it is important to practice good oral hygiene with brushing and flossing and regular dental appointments. If dry mouth is a problem for the Parkinson's disease patient, stimulating the flow of saliva by chewing on sour candy, sugarless gum, or ice cubes is helpful. Restricting caffeine intake and increasing fluid (water) intake can also be beneficial for dry mouth. A humidifier in the home may help combat a dry climate and dry mouth.

Vision

Dry eyes is a common complaint from Parkinson's disease patients. It is known that the automatic blink reflex is decreased in Parkinson's disease, resulting in tired, red, itchy dry eyes. Artificial tears may be helpful used two to three times a day.

Some patients may note blurred vision or difficulty adjusting vision to varying levels of light. These may be side effects of medication or they may be a change in vision. A visit to the eye doctor is recommended to rule out vision changes such as cataracts. Report these effects to the physician.

Medication

When treating Parkinson's disease, one of the initial steps is to take medication as prescribed by a physician. It is always beneficial to be as educated as possible about the medications prescribed. Physicians, nurses, and pharmacists are excellent resource persons for information on medication uses and side effects. The medications given for Parkinson's disease all have an impact on the amount of dopamine available for use by the brain. Please refer to chapter 1, "Diagnosis and Treatment," for more information on the current medical treatments for Parkinson's disease.

When beginning treatment with Parkinson's disease medications, there will be little improvement in symptoms the first few days. After a week of medication, however, there should be a noticeable change in slowness, rigidity, and/or tremor. If adequate changes are not noted, the Parkinson's disease patient or caregiver should contact the physician who prescribed the medication. Improvements may continue to be noted up to six months after initiation of drug treatment.

There can be interactions between different medications when prescribed and taken together; therefore, the Parkinson's disease patient or caregiver must keep records of medication taken. A good idea is to make a list of all medications taken, including the name, dosage, number of times taken during the day, and reason for taking the medication. Take this list to all physician visits and be sure the nurse makes a note or a copy of them. Update the list each time a change in medication is made.

If a patient has difficulty remembering to take medication or recalling if the medication has been taken, there are a few simple strategies to assist the patient or caregiver. A pill box can be purchased to divide out the doses of medication. Pill boxes can be small for daily dosing or large enough for a week's worth of medication doses. Shop for the pill box that best suits the patient's needs. Setting an alarm often helps patients remember to take a dose of medication. This can be a simple alarm on a wrist watch or an alarm made to be carried in the purse or pocket. The caregiver may be responsible for dispensing drugs for the more confused patient. It is important for the caregiver to be aware of medications and dosages because an overdose of medication can be quite detrimental to the patient and may end in hospitalization.

An illness or hospitalization may result in Parkinson's disease medications being discontinued for a period of time. Be aware that Parkinson's disease symptoms may worsen during this time; however, they should subside once treatment is resumed. Surgery for any patient usually requires that no food, water, or medication be taken after midnight before the surgery. Advise the physician about Parkinson's disease medications taken. It may be necessary for the patient's mobility for a dose of medication to be taken the morning of the surgery; otherwise, an admission to the hospital the night prior to surgery may be necessary.

Look for a pharmacist and pharmacy that one trusts. Getting the best prices for medications is important to Parkinson's disease patients, but it may be more beneficial to have a reliable pharmacist to turn to for information on medications, one who will have the patient's best interests in mind. Using a single pharmacy decreases the likelihood of contraindicated medications being dispensed or mistakes made when filling a prescription.

Sex

Sexual problems between Parkinson's disease patients and their spouses is a complaint that should be mentioned to a physician but is often not talked about. Medications can be the reason for a decrease in sexual desire. A review of the medications is a simple step to determining if the problem can be alleviated. An underlying depression may contribute to sexual dysfunction. Since depression is a common occurrence in Parkinson's disease, a neurologist may treat the depression with medication or may refer the patient to a psychologist or sex therapist. Complaints of impotence (inability to achieve and/or maintain an erection) are also noted in patients with Parkinson's disease. A referral to a urologist may be needed for a thorough examination to determine if there is another underlying cause for this. Medications are now available for impotence and can be prescribed by a physician. Please refer to chapter 8, "Sexuality and Parkinson's Disease," for further discussion.

Sleep

The Parkinson's disease patient may notice difficulties in initiating and maintaining sleep. Chapter 5, "Parkinson's Disease and Its Impact on Sleep," discusses sleep problems encountered in Parkinson's disease. Report any changes in sleep pattern or difficulties with sleep to a physician. A sleep disturbance can contribute to an overall change in Parkinson's disease symptoms for the patient. Vivid dreaming can especially hinder sleep if the dreams are troublesome or frightening to the patient. This usually is a side effect of medications and can frequently be relieved after review and change in dosing.

General Tips for Living with Parkinson's Disease

- It is always beneficial to have a telephone within reach. A cordless telephone is an excellent choice to carry from room to room to avoid having to "run" to answer a phone call. A telephone at waist level is also beneficial. It is much easier to reach for a phone at waist height than a phone mounted on the wall. And if a fall occurs and help is needed, it is much easier to reach a phone sitting on a table.
- An answering machine for the telephone is also a wise choice. Set the machine for the fourth or fifth ring so that it can be answered if possible. However, if it is not possible to get to the ringing phone, rather than risk a fall, let the machine take the message. One can then return the phone call at a convenient time.
- If it is difficult to hold the receiver of a phone, a speaker phone allows you to enjoy a conversation.
- Remote controls for television and lights can decrease the amount of maneuvering you have to do when relaxing.
- When shopping, make a list before you go and, if possible, make the list in the order you find products in the store. You can divide the items into categories such as meat, dairy, produce, bread, canned goods, paper, cleaning products, etc. Shop during the off hours to avoid crowds. Call stores beforehand to make sure they have the item you are looking for. Ask the store clerk to hold the item at the front of the store for you to avoid maneuvering in large department stores.
- Use stores that have drive-up facilities—for example, dry cleaners and pharmacies.

- Partially make out checks before you leave the house. Use credit cards for purchases and pay the monthly amount by writing one check only. Fold dollar bills in half in your wallet for easier access to get them out of your wallet or pocket.
- Always attempt to allow extra time for activities to prevent the stress and anxiety of being rushed.
- Check with your children, grandchildren, or neighborhood children for assistance with jobs around the house. Yard work, unloading groceries, and housecleaning are some examples of jobs that children and teenagers may do for a little extra spending money.
- The heat of the summer can be detrimental to Parkinson's disease patients. Some medications can increase the chance of suffering heat-related problems. Some Parkinson's disease patients tend to have heavy perspiration regardless of air temperature; therefore, being subjected to high temperatures and the sun can lead to the body's internal air-conditioning system not working efficiently. During the hot months of the year, attempt to cut back on strenuous activities or do them at the coolest times of the day. Drink plenty of fluids to avoid dehydration (at least 8 to 10 glasses of water a day). Wear light-weight, light-colored, loose-fitting clothing. Stay in air-conditioned buildings during the hottest part of the day. When outdoors, stay in the shade if possible. Avoid getting sunburned.

Summary

The ever-changing nature of Parkinson's disease presents challenges for patients, families, and the clinical care team. Communication, education, and persistence are often needed to solve the problems the parkinsonian faces every day. Resolution can be time-consuming, but with diligence the answers can be found. At times it may seem that just as one problem becomes manageable, another might step to the fore. It is at those times that the "Parki team" must again move into action. Parkinson's disease patients (and family members) have a duty to be informed about the disease and its many treatment options. Read materials, attend support group meetings, and participate in local Parkinson symposia to keep up with the latest news in research and self-help techniques. In these times of managed care, it is critical to stay active and involved in all aspects of health care. The health care team can be a vital resource for any person dealing with the everyday challenges associated with Parkinson's disease, but the most important member of the team is the parkinsonian. Take hold of the future!

7

Occupational and Physical Therapy

Britt Allen, Kristi F. Bennett, and Ginah S. Vrooman

Parkinson's disease symptoms have primarily been addressed through the use of medication, but there are many symptoms and manifestations of the disease that may be managed through the use of rehabilitation. Medications do help alleviate the primary physical manifestations that include stiffness (rigidity), slowness of movement (bradykinesia), and tremors or shaking of the hands. As the disease progresses, more and more daily activities are affected.[1] Physical, emotional, and social limitations appear and progress as the disease advances. Physical and occupational therapies can play a role in preventing or slowing the limitations associated with the advancement of Parkinson's disease. Increasingly, research has shown that with appropriate therapy, individuals with Parkinson's disease may be able to function more safely and independently.[2-6]

The idea of improvement through training and stimulation from therapists, caregivers, and family is both exciting and promising. Each individual with Parkinson's disease will respond differently to treatment. Trained occupational and physical therapists are important in determining which form of training is most needed by each individual. For the sake of clarification, we will discuss the characteristics and treatments of Parkinson's disease based on common clinical findings. We will look at the disease through three progressive stages—early, middle, and late—to provide a framework for treatment for individuals with Parkinson's disease.

EARLY STAGE THERAPY

The early stage of Parkinson's disease is commonly characterized by specific physical changes. Individuals rarely complain of a significant loss of independence or ability to perform day-to-day activities, but may report shaking of one hand while at rest, weakness in one leg, or tightness in the hip region.[7-8] Postural changes are also common. Hallmarks are a progressive stooped posture and forward rolling shoulders.[9] Additionally, individuals may begin to notice a decrease in handwriting skills or other fine motor activities.

TREATMENT

Physical and occupational therapy interventions in the early stage of Parkinson's disease focus primarily on education of affected individuals and their caregivers. Establishing a home exercise program should be an integral part of this education. Other concerns of individuals with Parkinson's disease and their caregivers may be addressed through community support services to relieve stress and enhance mental health. Depression is common with Parkinson's disease patients, and their caregivers can be affected by it as well.[8] Involvement in a support group or group therapy promotes socialization and comfort for both the patient and caregiver.[8,10-13] Physical and occupational therapists specialize in the physical activity concerns while trying to incorporate activities to address mental and social well-being.

Physical and occupational therapists educate Parkinson's disease patients and their caregivers according to the severity of the disease and individual capabilities. Education by a physical or occupational therapist typically consists of discussions and demonstrations of therapy goals with the patient and caregiver. A written home exercise program is provided, and specifics of the program are covered in detail. The home exercise program consists of exercises designed to prevent or delay the physical changes brought on by the disease. This exercise regimen should be done for approximately 15 to 20 minutes but may vary among individuals. Exercise should be challenging but should never cause pain. Home exercise programs usually include stretching, strengthening, and endurance exercises. (An example of a home exercise program can be found in Appendix A.) Each patient has different capabilities and should follow an individualized exercise program designed by a physical or occupational therapist.

Stretching exercises help increase muscle and joint flexibility and attempt to correct stooped posture. It is important to hold each stretch for 15 to 30 seconds in order to feel the stretching of the muscles and ligaments. Stretching exercises should be done daily, performing 1 to 3 repetitions of each stretch in a slow and controlled manner. The exercise routine should always *start* and *end* with stretching exercises, as it aids in warming up and cooling down muscles.

After stretching exercises to warm up the muscles, the next step is to begin strengthening exercises to enhance balance, posture, transfers, and gait stability. Studies show that back muscles (trunk extensors) are the first to show weakness in the early stage of Parkinson's disease.[4,8,14,15] Weak back muscles are usually evidenced by patients having flexed or bent backs. Emphasis is given to the extensor (straightening) muscles of the arms, trunk, and legs to correct the stooped posture. Strengthening exercises can be maximized by performing them in a standing position. Exercises to increase strength typically involve the use of cuff weights, dowel rods, or Theraband for resistance. The patient should breathe normally during the exercises and rest between exercises to prevent fatigue.

Endurance exercises are necessary to limit the decrease in cardiopulmonary (heart and lung) function that comes with natural aging. Individuals with Parkinson's disease are especially at risk of decreased heart and lung function due to decreased mobility and activity level. The best way to increase cardiopulmonary function is to stay active. Activities that help maintain or increase activity levels include walking laps (indoor or outdoor), walking on a treadmill, or pedaling a stationary bike. Each of these activities should be performed for 15 to 20 minutes at least three times a week. Appropriate footwear is recommended when doing exercises or when walking. Footwear should be comfortable and supportive. Low-heeled, crepe-soled shoes that are either slip-on or lace-up are best.[16]

PERSONAL CARE

Activities of daily living (ADLs) may be carried out without adaptive devices or assistance from a caregiver during the early stages of Parkinson's disease.[8] However, receiving proper advice and education from a physician or therapist on coping with changing physical and cognitive abilities may be beneficial. The therapist can also make suggestions for modifications or techniques to maintain family, leisure, and/or work roles. Explore activities that encourage fine motor control, coordination, and concentration. Examples include learning a new card game, doing word puzzles, or gardening. Early stage Parkinson's disease is also a good time to establish a scheduled exercise program along with regular daily activities. It may also be of benefit to plan daily walks, renew efforts at previously learned sports, or schedule recreational exercise like swimming and dancing. Additional information from books, pamphlets, physicians, and therapists on how the disease will affect lifestyle is available.

MIDDLE STAGE THERAPY

The middle stage of Parkinson's disease is characterized by worsening of symptoms.[7-9] The resting tremor increases and starts to affect many fine motor skills such as writing, fastening buttons, or manipulating knobs. In addition to an increased tremor, other physical changes such as bradykinesia, increased rigidity, and lack of coordination make daily tasks much more challenging. Individuals in this stage may still perform most daily tasks independently, but begin to require more assistance and assistive devices or activity modification. The role of the occupational and physical therapist is essential in helping the patient maintain independence and autonomy.

Personal care and grooming during this stage may be successfully addressed with proper techniques. Postural deviations may increase or show a worsening as well, characterized by a stooped, forward posture. During the middle stage of Parkinson's disease, individuals may develop problems initiating a movement or making a change in movement.[2,5,18,19] This is especially true during walking and is one of the most challenging symptoms for individuals with Parkinson's disease. Additional gait characteristics seen in individuals with Parkinson's disease include a shuffling of the feet, lack of ability to turn, poor arm swing, freezing, and lack of ability to weight shift.[19] Along with these deviations, a forward-bent posture increases the likelihood of falling forward while attempting to walk or to change directions. During the middle stage, a decline of motor planning may develop. Some individuals with middle stage Parkinson's disease are challenged if performing a task that requires several steps, and tend to have difficulty with concentrating on more than one task at a time.

In the middle stage, therapy interventions are divided into two parts: corrective and compensatory therapy programs.

Corrective Therapy

Corrective therapy exercise programs attempt to counter the physical limitations that Parkinson's disease imposes on patients. This program attempts to increase general strength, restore upright posture, and improve balance and coordination. Appendix A includes illustrations for the following exercises.

Strength and Endurance. General strengthening and endurance exercises attempt to restore or maintain active range of motion for the arms and legs. "Active range of motion" means that the patient can move his or her limbs actively through the full range of motion without any assistance. Some individuals in the middle stage of Parkinson's disease may need to devote careful attention to performing exercises through the full range of motion. Patients who can perform active range of motion exercises should begin with progressive resistive exercises which involve the use of some form of resistance, such as dumbbells, cuff weights, or Theraband. Individuals in this stage should also perform the same endurance exercises recommended in the early stage, such as walking or stationary bicycling.

Postural training includes trunk elongation, pelvic mobilization, pelvic and shoulder separation and rotation, and strengthening of the back extensor muscles. Trunk elongation stretches the side muscles of the trunk. It is performed by reaching one arm overhead toward the opposite side while sitting upright in a chair. This causes lengthening of muscles on one side of the trunk and shortening on the other side. Pelvic mobilization, also called pelvic tilting, is best done while sitting at the edge of the chair or bed with feet flat on the floor or in a standing position. Pelvic mobilization is a specialized technique included in skilled physical and occupational therapy treatment. Pelvic and shoulder separation and rotation are required for the natural movement of walking. The lower part of the body (hips and legs) is synchronous with the upper body (shoulders and arms) when walking. Exercise for separation involves pendulum-like exercises with the right arm and left leg moving simultaneously, and the left arm and right leg also moving in rhythm. These activities can be performed standing, sitting, or lying down. Strengthening exercises for the back extensors attempt to correct the stooped posture that is common in Parkinson's disease. These exercises can be done lying on your stomach or standing with your arms at your side using a dowel rod or Theraband.

Balance and Coordination. Balance and coordination exercises include sitting and standing activities, as well as training to correct gait pattern deviations. Sitting and standing activities focus on increasing the individual's ability to independently perform activities of daily living.[24] Sitting activities involve reaching and weight shifting. These activities simulate activities such as putting on one's shoes, getting out of a chair, and repositioning onerself in a chair. Standing activities involve increasing the base of support for dynamic standing and static standing tolerance while carrying out functional activities such as kitchen chores. Dynamic standing activities include reaching and bending with proper body mechanics for placing items in cabinets or in overhead closets and picking items up from the floor. Shifting weight from side to side and forward and backward are gait preparation exercises which aid in transitioning body weight during the stance and swing phases of walking.

Not all gait problems are caused by balance or coordination deficits.[25] For this reason, training to correct actual gait pattern deviations is also utilized. Heel-toe raises and toe tapping encourage heel strike for a "heel-toe" walking pattern and are performed in both sitting and standing positions. Gait deviations are effectively addressed utilizing specialized techniques and proper education of the patient.[1,8,10,13,19] Training in negotiating obstacles can enhance reflex reactions and encourage safe handling of the environment where obstructions on the floor or on the walkway may be found. It is recommended for people with Parkinson's disease to make turns widely, in a big "U-turn" manner, to decrease the occurrence of shuffling and freezing (inability to move out of a position) which might contribute to a fall. To overcome the obstructions in their pathways safely, patients should be trained to look far ahead and plan their moves in advance.

When going up steps or stepping onto a curb, always lead with the stronger leg. When going down steps or stepping off of curbs, lead with the weaker leg. Always use siderails or handholds if available. When following these instructions, remember to position yourself as close to the step or curb as possible and take one step at a time. If using an assistive device, the device should lead the movement and be placed where you are stepping. Training for walking on different types of terrain (level and uneven surfaces such as ramps, steps, and curbs) with and without assistive devices is incorporated in skilled treatment.

Postural Reflexes. Postural righting reflexes are used to regain and correct balance to prevent falls. Individuals with Parkinson's disease exhibit decreased postural righting reflexes. This is caused by the stiffness (rigidity), slowness of movement (bradykinesia), and difficulty initiating a movement (akinesia) experienced by Parkinson's disease patients.[6,7,13,19–21] Exercises to maximize postural righting reflexes include walking sideways, tandem walking (walking on a straight line), marching, braiding (feet crossing over), and walking backward. All activities should be performed with supervision and support as needed for safety.

Fine Motor Control. Fine motor coordination needs to be addressed and can be improved through occupational therapy by increasing hand strength, dexterity or flexibility, and control.[2,18,20,22–27] Wrist, hand, and finger exercises and stretches are prescribed and proper techniques taught by the therapist. Repetitive exercise and activity requiring rhythmical and accurate movements can help to improve the graded movement needed for fine motor skills.[5,8,18,20] Manipulating small objects in the hands helps improve flexibility, an essential skill.[2,25,26] Rigidity and tremor may impact fine motor skills to the extent that adaptive equipment is required. Proper instruction and training on the use of adaptive equipment for dressing, grooming, and other everyday activities are provided, along with exercise and activities to improve fine motor coordination, during occupational therapy.

Compensatory Therapy Program

Compensatory therapy includes energy conservation techniques, breathing exercises, transfer and transition training, bed mobility training, and gait training with or without the use of an assistive device.

Energy Conservation. Energy conservation techniques help manage fatigue by teaching the patient to rest between tasks or during the task as needed. Breaking a task into smaller sections with planned rest breaks provides an opportunity to perform a rather involved task without excessive fatigue. Using proper body mechanics for lifting and carrying objects is also a means of conserving energy. Energy conservation techniques are not specific to Parkinson's disease patients and are also good techniques for caregivers and other family members to adopt.

Relaxation Techniques. Deep-breathing exercises are an excellent means of relaxation. They are also useful to improve rigid trunk muscles which limit the chest expansion ability of the individual. These exercises primarily involve inhaling through the nose and exhaling through the mouth. One should concentrate on breathing during inhalation and contracting the abdomen slowly on exhalation. Good breathing techniques facilitate louder vocalization and longer sentences when speaking. Decreased breathing rates also help decrease overall body fatigue and allow relaxation.

Transfer and Transition Training. Transfer and transition training is a necessity for safe home mobility. Typical transfers include sit-to-stand, chair-to-chair, and chair-to-bed transfers.

Sit-to stand. In the sit-to-stand process, the proper positioning and sequence should be:

(1) Scoot buttocks toward the edge of the chair *(photo 1)*.
(2) Arrange feet flat on the floor, angled slightly behind knees *(photo 2)*.
(3) Lean forward with "nose over the toes" and shift the body weight in a forward and upward motion *(photo 3)*.
(4) Straighten your knees looking ahead and keeping the shoulders back *(photo 4)*.

Chair-to-bed or chair-to-chair transfers require the sit-to-stand transition first. Once standing, the patient should follow the following process:

(1) Turn the heels toward the bed or chair to transfer to.
(2) Step back until the edge of the bed or chair is felt behind the knees.
(3) Reach back for the surface (for safety) and then slowly lower to a sitting position by bending the knees.

Remember to bend slightly forward when sitting to help maintain balance and control the transfer.

Bed mobility. Bed mobility training may or may not be required for individuals in this stage of the disease process. Often, poor mobility techniques are begun during this stage due to rigidity and poor motor control. The result of these compensations is usually ineffective and awkward bed mobility. Proper techniques can be taught by occupational and physical therapists, with simple energy conservation techniques being emphasized. For example, sit-to-lying motor preparations and positioning should involve three steps:

1. Sit at the edge of the bed *(photo 5)*.
2. Lower the upper body down toward the head of the bed with hand flat on the bed, while simultaneously lifting the legs up onto the bed to come to a sidelying position *(photos 6, 7, and 8)*.
3. Roll onto the back, keeping the entire body straight *(photos 9 and 10)*.

Sitting up from the lying position should be performed in the following fashion:

1. Scoot to the edge of the bed and bend both knees.

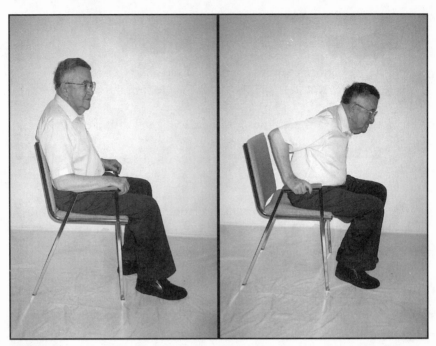

Photo 1   Photo 2

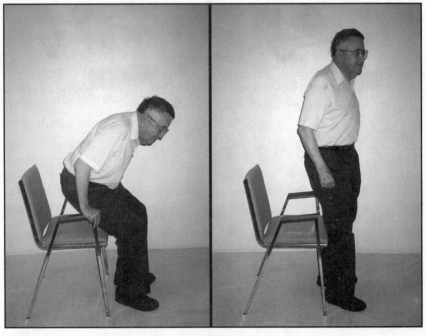

Photo 3   Photo 4

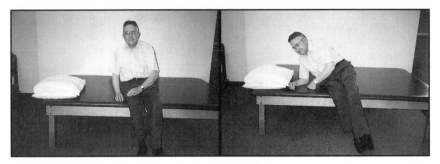

Photo 5 Photo 6

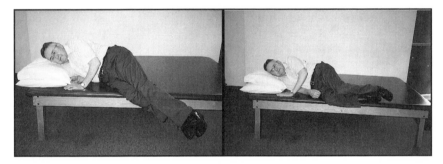

Photo 7 Photo 8

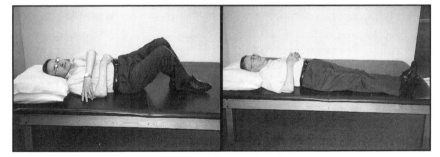

Photo 9 Photo 10

2. Roll onto your side facing the edge of the bed while keeping your knees bent.
3. Lower both legs off of the bed while pushing with the arms to sit up.

Gait Training. Gait training during the middle stage of the disease process may include the addition of an assistive device to manage freezing and prevent falls.[28-30] Assistive devices commonly used for individuals with Parkinson's disease are canes and walkers. Proper training and fitting should be provided by a physical or occupational therapist to ensure safe and effective use of the device. *Canes* provide the least support but are ideal for patients who are fully weight-bearing yet need some assistance with balance due to weak muscles of the legs *(photo 11)*. The height of the cane should be level with the hipbone and allow the hand to rest with the elbow bent at a 20- to 30-degree angle. Different types of canes include straight canes that are wooden or adjustable aluminum, walking sticks or staffs that help in walking upright and tall, and step-over wands that have a release button to help initiate a step when freezing occurs during walking. *Walkers* provide a wider and more stable base of support *(photo 12)*. They may be prescribed for patients requiring moderate to maximum assistance with balance and coordination during ambulation. For people with Parkinson's disease, a rolling walker is easier to use due to the freezing phenomenon. Rolling walkers also make the mental sequencing required for walking less complex. The walkers may be divided into the conventional two-wheeled walker with the wheels on the front of the walker *(photo 13)*, a three-wheeled walker *(photo 14)*, and a four-wheeled walker. Most of these rolling walkers have hand-controlled brakes, and many have a seat or a basket that can be added.

Personal Care

Throughout the progression of Parkinson's disease, activities of daily living such as dressing, bathing or showering, grooming, toileting, eating, and drinking are influenced by the changes created by the disease. Rigidity, tremors, bradykinesia, and akinesia impact these activities differently for each individual in various degrees of impaired coordination, control, and flexibility.[8] An occupational therapist can prescribe the appropriate adaptive equipment and teach strategies using the equipment to enable those with Parkinson's disease to perform daily acitivities with greater independence. Taking the necessary measures to ensure independence and improved

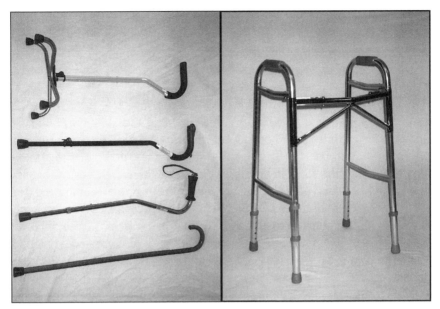

Photo 11

Photo 12

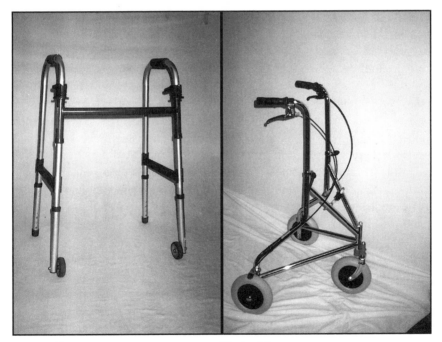

Photo 13

Photo 14

safety can be complicated by an individual's need for control and refusal to "give into" the disease. It must be acknowledged that compensating for deficits does not mean giving up. Accepting the use of adaptive equipment and using techniques and strategies to perform activities safely and efficiently is necessary as Parkinson's disease progresses.

To maintain quality of life during the middle stage of Parkinson's disease, continuing an active lifestyle that includes socialization, hobbies, and regular exercise will become increasingly important.[22,25–27,31] Muscle tightness and/or decreased range of motion may make reaching and bending more difficult. Slower, less coordinated movements of the arms and legs interfere with precise and accurate movements required for dressing. Manipulating small objects like fasteners and carrying out large rhythmical movements like brushing teeth or hair may be affected. However, with adaptive devices, home modifications, and energy conservation techniques, activities of daily living may be performed with little or no assistance from a caregiver. Although some tasks may take longer for the individual to complete, emphasis should be placed on the ability to complete tasks.

Dressing. An individual's choice of what to wear is important to self-esteem, dignity, and comfort. If one's preferences are for clothing which enable safe and independent dressing and undressing, modifications will not need to be made. However, as Parkinson's disease progresses, preferred clothing or dressing techniques could hinder independence or safety.[27] If safety is compromised, different clothing options or use of adaptive equipment may become necessary. One simple change is to dress and undress while in a seated position to decrease the chance of falls. Standing should only be done to raise trousers. Dressing while seated will also help to conserve energy.

Bradykinesia and akinesia often result in limited coordination, especially in the upper extremities. Lack of coordination often causes difficulty with fasteners such as buttons and hooks on clothing. Shirts and pants will be easier to take on and off with front closures, preferably zippers and/or large buttons that can be easily distinguished from the fabric. If there are buttons, a button hook with an enlarged handle can be helpful. Button hooks as well as other assistive devices discussed can be purchased from medical supply stores or medical supply catalogs. For clothing with zippers, a zipper pull (large loop placed on zippers) can also help by creating a larger area to grasp. A zipper pull may also be used by placing the thumb into the loop when decreased range of motion, tremor, or arthritis is present. Velcro fasteners can be attached under buttons or for closings on skirts or slacks for even easier dressing.

Dressing for the Parkinson's disease patient with bradykinesia may also be made easier by dressing to rhythmic music.[6] Visual stimulation provided by dressing in front of a mirror may also be helpful.[6] Still others find that verbally instructing themselves as they dress helps speed the dressing process.[5,9] Retrieving all items needed at once and laying them out in order can conserve energy by eliminating the need to stand up and sit down several times during the dressing process. This technique also helps one to sequence items for dressing.

A dressing stick or reacher can be used when retrieving articles of clothing that are out of reach, as well as pushing and pulling garments off and on the legs or over the head. Reachers can also be used to remove clothing from hangers, arrange clothing, and pick up socks, shoes, and other items from the floor or shelves. A dressing stick or reacher is especially important if an individual has rigidity or decreased range of motion in the arms, neck, and trunk.

Pullover shirt styles and pants with elastic waistbands may also make dressing more efficient. Lightweight, stretchy fabrics will also enhance comfort. Slip-on shoes or shoes with elastic shoelaces that do not have to be untied will require less energy to put on and take off. A long-handled shoehorn and a sock aide are used to put on shoes and socks while seated. These modifications will lessen the amount of bending that can result in increased dizziness, and will also help to compensate for impaired sitting balance.

Grooming. Activities such as combing or brushing hair, brushing teeth, shaving, and applying make-up should be performed independently by an individual with Parkinson's disease for as long as possible. Everyday activities such as these encourage movement, coordination, dexterity, self-esteem, and dignity, as well as enabling individuals to retain control over their appearance. Adaptive techniques and devices can prolong the ability to carry out these tasks with greater ease.

Accurate or graded movements, such as those required when reaching for an object, may become increasingly difficult as the middle stage of Parkinson's disease progresses. Items that are used frequently should be kept within easy reach. These items may be placed on an anti-slip pad so they can be grasped without knocking them over. Electric devices like an electric toothbrush or razor allow tasks to be performed efficiently while conserving energy. It is best to "pace" activities of daily living by simplifying the task or by breaking the task down into steps and sitting periodically. Standing while performing all grooming tasks may increase dizziness or result in unnecessary fatigue.

Weighted handles on utensils and assistive devices help compensate for tremors and give the user a greater sense of where the device is being moved. Long-handled equipment may be used if reaching backward or toward the feet has become difficult due to decreased range of motion or flexibility in the elbows, wrists, and shoulders. Enlarged grips are used if there is decreased dexterity in the hands. For instance, a hairbrush may need an extended handle with an enlarged grip for an individual with Parkinson's disease to effectively reach overhead and brush his or her hair.

Bathing/Showering. Utilizing the proper equipment and using it correctly can reduce falls, facilitate safe transfers, and maximize independence. An occupational therapist can assist in determining what equipment is appropriate for each individual and provide instruction on correct installation and efficient use. It is also important to simplify the bathroom by removing unnecessary items. For instance, all throw rugs should be removed from the bathroom (and all other rooms) to prevent tripping. Waxed floor surfaces can also cause falls and should be left unwaxed.

Specialized equipment can make the bathroom safer for the Parkinson's patient. Strategically placed grab bars increase the safety of transferring in and out of the bathtub or shower. Adhesive nonslip strips or a non-slip bathmat may help prevent slipping when transferring in and out of the tub or shower. An extended, hand-held shower hose can be utilized to limit the amount of turning required when standing. If standing while bathing or if transferring in and out of the tub or shower becomes too difficult, a shower chair is essential. Transferring in and out of the shower can be simplified and made much safer with the use of a shower chair *(photo 15)*. It also eliminates excessive standing by showering in a

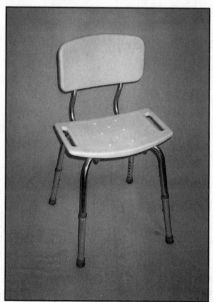

seated position using an extended shower hose. The use of a long-handled bath sponge can help individuals with impaired movement maintain a level of independence by allowing them to reach their back and feet. A wash mitt can be secured to an individual's wrist if tremor or impaired coordination interferes with bathing.

Toileting. Standing from or sitting on a standard toilet may become difficult due to muscle rigidity, weakness, and impaired coordination of movement. Utilizing adaptive equipment, like an elevated toilet seat with arm rails or grab bars, can ensure safety and enable independence with toileting.

Photo 15

Space in the bathroom should be adequate for assistive devices, such as a walker, to be easily maneuvered within the bathroom for correct transfers to and from the toilet. It is also important to reduce excessive bending or turning while toileting by placing the toilet-paper holder within reach. If tearing off the required amount of paper is troublesome due to impaired muscle control, single sheets of toilet paper or a paper dispenser may help. Keeping the light on in the bathroom or using night-lights will also help to prevent falls by enabling the individual to find his or her way after dark. Frequent toileting during the night may warrant a bedside commode to reduce the risk of falls

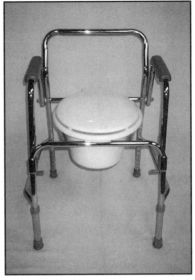

Photo 16

(photo 16). This device will also allow more time for sleep by decreasing the distance to a commode.

Eating and Drinking. The ability to use utensils and get food items from plate to mouth is affected by both rigidity of the hand and wrist and slow pace. Techniques to alleviate early swallowing difficulties resulting from muscle rigidity should be applied as instructed in chapter 9, "Speech, Swallowing, and Communication." Adaptations to compensate for decreased movement and coordination may include an optimal sitting position (sitting straight in the chair and keeping the head and chin level), and utilizing enlarged, weighted grips on utensils to compensate for tremor. Wrist weights can also alleviate tremors for more controlled movements. Deep spoons or swivel spoons will reduce spillage.

Foods need to be cut into smaller pieces than usual so they can be safely chewed and swallowed. It is important for those with Parkinson's disease to be able to cut their own food easily. Sharp knives work best because they require less effort. Specialized knives, known as rocker knives, can be helpful to those with decreased range of motion. Plates and bowls with high sides will make scooping up foods easier, and antislip pads or surfaces will prevent the dish from slipping. As feeding difficulties increase, further advice should be obtained from an occupational or speech therapist.

Handwriting. Handwriting of people with Parkinson's disease often becomes very small. This is referred to as micrographia. The handwriting may also become difficult to read or illegible due to decreased dexterity, tremor, and perceptual difficulties. Maintaining good posture and supporting both arms on a stable writing surface is required. The nondominant hand may be used to stabilize the writing hand at the wrist if necessary. A pen grip or a piece of foam placed around a pen may be useful. Weighted pens can also be used to dampen tremor. Felt-tip pens may be easier to use than other types. If the handwiting becomes smaller as one writes, the writer should stop, exercise the arm a moment, and begin writing again. Writing programs like Callirobics are designed to improve fine motor coordination and control through repetition.[32]

Communication. Difficulties using the telephone usually center around dialing numbers and communicating loudly enough while holding the receiver. Gooseneck receiver holders can be clamped to a tabletop to eliminate the need for sustained holding, or a speaker phone can be used. Many phone companies provide these special phones as a free service for those with difficulty manipulating standard equipment.[27] Telephones with large punch-button numbers and memory buttons so phone numbers can be easily retrieved can be very helpful. Amplifiers for the earpiece and mouthpiece are also available in a variety of amplifications and sizes.

Emergency alarms that can be worn around the neck as a pendant or on the wrist as a bracelet are indispensable items to people with Parkinson's disease in the case of falls or other accidents. These alarms are best employed in conjunction with a telephone equipped with memory so emergency numbers and caregivers' numbers can be dialed quickly. When placing phones in the home, make sure they are on a low table that can be easily reached from the floor. It is helpful to place a chair next to the phone to prevent excessive standing.

In addition to these treatments for the physical impairments of Parkinson's disease, it is important to keep in mind that mental and emotional states may also be affected. It is therefore necessary to start training a family member or caregiver as soon as therapy is initiated. Repetitions and consistency are vital to the effectiveness of therapy. Caregivers should reinforce what the patient is able to do to help maintain a sense of control and to boost morale. Denial may be magnified during this stage of the disease process. Emotional support from therapists, physician, and caregivers can help tremendously with coping. Group therapy is very important in decreasing apprehension and increasing self-assurance by encouraging socialization and continued interactions with others.

LATE STAGE THERAPY

The late stages of Parkinson's disease are characterized by progressively worsening symptoms that may prevent the patient from living alone or without assistance. Supervision and assistance for activities of daily living may be required. Tremor may diminish in this stage, but rigidity and bradykinesia are quite marked. Bed mobility and transfers are performed with great difficulty or are not possible without assistance. The flexed posture experienced by the person with Parkinson's disease also makes most tasks difficult because the needed range of motion is not available. Ambulation may still be possible, but the gait pattern is very slow and shuffling of the feet makes it ineffective. Extreme balance and coordination deficits make sitting and standing without support dangerous. As the disease progresses, most of the waking hours are spent in bed or in a wheelchair, which may be uncomfortable or hard to maintain due to postural deficits.

Treatment

During the late stage of Parkinson's disease, education again takes on great importance. Safety of the patient is essential, but equally important is the safety of the caregiver. Individuals with Parkinson's disease during this stage require assistance, and if the caregiver's health is compromised, so is the ability to provide needed assistance. Some important training recommendations for the caregiver include proper body mechanics, pressure relief techniques, wheelchair management and mobility, bed positioning, and passive range of motion exercises.

A wheelchair is a good piece of equipment to have if falls become more frequent. A wheelchair may become a necessity if balance is very poor when standing or ambulation is very unstable. The wheelchair helps to minimize the frequency of falls, reducing the risks of major injuries resulting from a fall. Appropriate recommendations and wheelchair measurements should be provided by a therapist. As with any new piece of equipment, the patient and caregiver should receive proper training on wheelchair use and safety. This training should include the manipulations and management of the wheelchair, preparations and positioning of the wheelchair for transfers, and wheelchair mobility for both indoor and outdoor activities (i.e., ramps and curbs as well as level surfaces).

Both the patient and the caregiver should be educated on the parts of the wheelchair and proper manipulation of the brakes and footrests, both for safety and in preparation for transfers. Wheelchair management and mobility are essential for energy conservation, safety of both patient and caregiver, and ease of movement through home or in the community. When preparing for transfers out of or into a wheelchair, the chair should be placed at a 45-degree angle next to the surface to transfer to or from (bed or toilet seat). Lock the chair in place, then remove the armrest and footrest, if possible. The person with Parkinson's disease should then transfer as previously described in the section on middle stage treatment, with assistance provided as needed by the caregiver. When propelling a wheelchair, the patient should use both arms. If the patient has good leg mobility, he or she may be able to "walk" the chair with his or her feet while propelling the chair with the arms. Proper techniques should be used when pushing a wheelchair up or down a curb and can be taught by either a physical or occupational therapist.

If an individual is wheelchair-bound, pressure relief techniques and frequent position changes should be used. Pressure relief techniques primarily involve placing the arms on the armrests and pushing down in order to lift the buttocks off the seat to relieve continuous pressure on tissues. Shifting weight from side to side every 15 to 30 minutes is also recommended. For individuals with more advanced Parkinson's disease, this may not be physically possible; for such persons, a customized seat cushion may be prescribed.

Position changes are also important when lying in bed. Bed positioning is therapeutic for weight-bearing and pressure relief to decrease the chances of bedsores and joint contractures. This is especially true for people with Parkinson's disease where decreased mobility can cause further, progressive debilitation. Bed positioning should be done in good comfort while maintaining joint integrity. Cushioning, such as a pillow, should be placed between the knees and ankles and between the arms when laying on your side *(photo 17)*. When laying on the back or stomach, appropriate cushioning for pressure relief should also be used *(photos 18 and 19)*.

Modifications should also be carefully considered for easy access to cabinets, closets, and tables throughout the home.[30] Positioning of furniture and door openings should be evaluated to insure ease of propelling a wheelchair throughout the home. All throw rugs should be removed from the home or secured to the floor to prevent tripping.

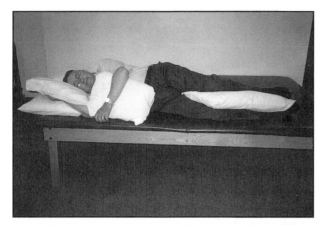

Photo 17. Sidelying

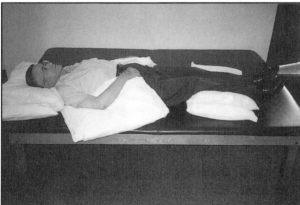

Photo 18. Supine

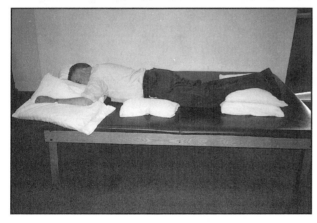

Photo 19. Prone

Exercise

Exercise and stretching become increasingly important in this stage because rigidity may increase, making it more difficult to be active and move about the environment. Maintaining existing movement and mobility should be reinforced to whatever degree possible in order to control an increase in rigidity. The caregiver can continue to participate in exercises, or a videotape can be used for persons with Parkinson's disease to follow on their own. Motor planning, simultaneous tasks, and following verbal or visual instructions may all become difficult for the patient. It is then necessary for the caregiver or health care professional to assist with an exercise by asking the individual to perform that particular exercise while gently guiding the movement of the limb.

These *passive range of motion exercises* are vital to musculoskeletal preservation during the advanced middle and late stages. These exercises involve moving an individual's arms and legs to stretch the muscles and maintain joint function. It is important to seek the advice of a physical or occupational therapist when performing passive range of motion exercises. A caregiver's hand placement should be close to the joint and bring the extremity to the end range as much as possible within the limits of pain. The exercises should be done in a slow and gentle manner. Perform 10 to 15 repetitions of each exercise at least twice daily with the patient sitting in a chair or lying on a bed.

The general aim of intervention throughout the later stages of Parkinson's disease is to modify and adapt lifestyle while still meeting the needs of the individual patient and caregiver. It remains important to continue appropriate hobbies and interests, but they may need to be modified. For example, gardening may be done in pots on a table, with brief standing or while sitting, rather than in the ground. Card games, board games, or crafts may need to be simplified or adapted to the capabilities of the person with Parkinson's disease. Specific suggestions for other hobbies and interests can be obtained from a therapist.

Parkinson's disease is a progressive disorder and the information outlined in this chapter will not stop the progression of the disease. Many agencies and organizations are available to support and help the family or caregiver as well as the patient. They may include support groups, respite care, assistance programs such as Meals on Wheels, and church organizations. Research continues to make strides in relaying positive outcomes for individuals with Parkinson's disease. Improved independence, increased activity level, increased community activity and socialization, and decreased feelings of hopelessness and helplessness are all addressed by the ideas and activities suggested in this chapter.

REFERENCES

1. Morris, M. E., Matayas, T. A., Iansek, R. and Summers, J. J. (1996). "Temporal stability of gait in Parkinson's disease." *Physical Therapy* 76(7):763.

2. Alberts, J. L., Tresilian, J. R., and Stelmach, G. E. (1998). "The co-ordination and phasing of bilateral prehension task: The influence of Parkinson's disease." *Brain* 121:725.

3. Day, B. L., Dick, J. R. P., and Marsden, C. D. (1984). "Patients with Parkinson's disease can employ a predictive motor strategy." *Journal of Neurology, Neurosurgery, and Psychiatry* 47:129.

4. Palmer, S. S., Mortimer, J. A., Webster, D. D., Bistevins, R., and Dickinson, G. L. (1986). "Exercise therapy for Parkinson's disease." *Archive of Physical Medicine and Rehabilitation* 67:741.

5. Praamstra, P., Stegeman, D. F., Cools, A. R., and Horstink, M. W. I. M. (1998). "Reliance on external cues for movement initiation in Parkinson's disease: Evidence from movement-related potentials." *Brain* 121:167.

6. Dibble, L. D., and Nicholson, D. E. (1997). "Sensory cueing improves motor performance and rehabilitation in persons with Parkinson's disease." *Neurology Report* 21(4):117.

7. Schenkman, M., and Butler, R. B. (1989). "A model for multi-system evaluation treatment of individuals with Parkinson's disease." *Physical Therapy* 69 (11):932.

8. Schenkman, M., and Butler, R. B. (1995). "Pharmacological and nonpharmacological interventions in the treatment of Parkinson's disease." *Physical Therapy* 75:363.

9. Parkinson's Outreach Program. (1997). *Resource and Home Exercise Manual.*

10. Morris, M. E., and Iansek, R. (1997). "Gait disorders in Parkinson's disease: A framework for physical therapy practice." *Neurology Report* 21(4):125.

11. Gauthier, L., Dalziel, S., and Gauthier, S. (1987). "The benefits of group occupational therapy for patients with Parkinson's disease." *American Journal of Occupational Therapy* 41(6):360.

12. Hunt, B. (1988). "Continuity of car maximizes autonomy of the elderly." *American Journal of Occupational Therapy* 42(6):392.

13. Szekely, B. C., Kosanovich, N. N., and Sheppard, W. (1982). "Adjunctive treatment in Parkinson's disease: Physical therapy and comprehensive group therapy." *Rehabilitation Literature* 43(3-4):72.

14. Smithson, F., Morris, M. E., and Iansek, R. (1998). "Performance on clinical tests of balance in Parkinson's disease." *Physical Therapy* 78(6):577.

15. Glendinning, D. (1997). "A rationale for strength training in patients with Parkinson's disease." *Neurology Report* 21(4):132.

16. Williams, F. T. (1985). *Rehabilitation in the Aging,* Second Edition. New York: Roman Press.

17. Bloxham, C. A., Mindel, T. A., and Frith, C. D. (1984). "Initiation and execution of predictable and unpredictable movements in Parkinson's disease." *Brain* 107:371.

18. Majsak, M. J., Kaminski, T., Gentile, A. M., and Flanagan, J. R. (1998). "The reaching movements of patients with Parkinson's disease under self-determined maximal speed and visually cued conditions." *Brain* 121:755.

19. Rogers, M. W. (1991). "Motor control problems in Parkinson's disease." In M. J. Lister, ed., *Contemporary Management of Motor Control Problems: Proceedings of the II Step Conference.* Alexandria, Va.: Foundation for Physical Therapy, Inc.

20. Platz, T., Brown, R. G., and Marsden, C. D. (1998). "Training improves the speed of aimed movements in Parkinson's disease." *Brain* 121:505.

21. Dietz, V., Berger, W., and Horstmann, G. A. (1988). "Posture in Parkinson's disease: Impairment of reflexes and programming." *Annals of Neurology* 24:660.

22. Cohen, Andrea M., and Weiner, W. J. (1994). *The Comprehensive Management of Parkinson's Disease.* New York: Demos Publications.

23. Calne, D. B. (1993). "Treatment of Parkinson's disease." *New England Journal of Medicine* 329:1021.

24. Pearce, J. M. S. (1992). *Parkinson's Disease and Its Management.* New York: Oxford University Press.

25. Pedretti, L. W. (1996). *Occupational Therapy Practice Skills for Physical Dysfunction.* St. Louis, Mo.: Mosby-Year Book, Inc.

26. Tramby, C. A. (1995). *Occupational Therapy for Physical Dysfunction.* Baltimore, Md.: Williams & Wilkins.

27. Turner, A., Foster, M., and Johnson, S. E. (1996). *Occupational Therapy and Physical Dysfunction: Principles, Skills, and Practice.* New York: Pearson Professional Limited.

28. Turnbull, G. I. (1992). *Clinics in Physical Therapy: Physical Therapy Management of Parkinson's Disease.* New York: Churchhill Livingstone Inc.

29. Lewis, C. B. (1989). *Improving Mobility in Older Persons: A Manual for Geriatric Specialists.* Maryland: Aspen Publishers.

30. Axtell, A. J., and Yosuda, Y. L. (1993). "Assistive devices and home modifications in geriatric rehabilitation." *Geriatric Rehabilitation* 9(4):803.

31. Davis, C. M. (1997). *Complementary Therapies in Rehabilitation.* Thorofore, N.J.: SLACK Incorporated.

32. Laufer, L. (1995). *Callirobics.* Charlottesville, Va.: Liora Laufer.

33. Weiner, W. J., and Singer, C. (1993). "Parkinson's disease and non-pharmacologic treatment programs." *Journal of the American Geriatrics Society* 37:359.

8

Sexuality and Parkinson's Disease

Lauren Seeberger

Human sexuality is a very complicated subject, involving both emotional and physical aspects. We have a certain need to be held and touched that cannot be met through other means. An important part of this fulfillment comes from sexual encounters. People with Parkinson's disease are known to have changes in their sexuality. Some of these relate to dysfunction of the nervous system, while others stem from changes in self-image and relationships.

BACKGROUND

Some 10 to 20 million men in the United States have impotence, which is defined as "lack of power" or specifically, in the male, an inability to achieve and sustain an erection. Most impotence arises from "organic" or physical causes, including medical illness or medications. Sometimes impotence is due to psychological causes such as depression, poor sex drive, or performance anxiety. Men with Parkinson's disease are twice as likely as men of the same age to have impotence. Not much is known about sexual dysfunction in women with Parkinson's disease since they are much less likely to report sexual problems. Women with Parkinson's disease have more difficulty with inhibitions, loss of libido, and poor arousal. They may also experience pain with sex due to vaginal tightness or dryness. Since much more is understood about the sexual function of men with Parkinson's disease, this chapter will primarily discuss evaluating and treating male impotence.

THE FIVE PHASES OF MALE SEXUAL RESPONSE

First phase: Libido—the sex drive.

Second phase: Erection—blood filling the penis and making it rigid.

Third phase: Orgasm—the climax of sexual excitement.

Fourth phase: Ejaculation—the release of seminal fluid.

Fifth phase: Refractory period—the time after ejaculation when stimulation is difficult.

Sexual dysfunction in men can happen during any one of the first four phases. The erection phase is extremely complex and relies on teamwork from the brain, blood vessels, nerves and hormones. Initially, the brain senses excitement and sends messages to different systems for erection to take place. The penis has spongy tissue with many blood vessels. Normally, the blood vessels are constricted (tight), but during sexual excitation chemical and nerve stimulation result in relaxation of the blood vessels. This permits the penis to fill with blood and become rigid enough for intercourse. Difficulty during this phase leads to erectile dysfunction.

ERECTILE DYSFUNCTION

Erectile dysfunction can be divided into organic (physical) and non-organic (psychological) causes. Physical causes of impotence are overwhelmingly the most common. The primary risk factors for organic impotence include medical diseases that cause blood-flow problems, such as diabetes mellitus, hypertension, and atherosclerosis. Chronic smoking and alcohol abuse may also lead to impotence. Those who have had pelvic vascular surgery or prostate or spinal-cord surgery are at risk for erectile dysfunction. Lastly, many types of medications may cause impotence as a side effect, such as those used to treat peptic ulcer disease, depression, and high blood pressure. You should check with your doctor if you have questions regarding a particular medication. For more details, see table 1.

Nonorganic erectile dysfunction results from many psychological

TABLE 1
RISK FACTORS FOR
ERECTILE DYSFUNCTION

* Medical history of:
    —Diabetes mellitus
    —Hypertension
    —Atherosclerosis
    —Chronic neurological disease
    —Smoking cigarettes
    —Alcohol abuse

* Surgical history including:
    —Prostatectomy
    —Pelvic vascular surgery
    —Spinal-cord injury or spinal-cord surgery

* Hormonal deficiency from:
    —Severe kidney or liver disease
    —Treatment of prostate cancer
    —Other causes

* Side effects of medications:
    —Peptic ulcer drugs
    —Blood pressure medications
    —Sedatives
    —Hormones
    —Cold and allergy preparations

---

factors. One is anxiety about being able to get and maintain an erection sufficient to perform the sexual act. Performance anxiety can be experienced by any man on occasion, but if it leads to frequent failures the worsening anxiety may cause impotence. Some men have a low libido while others may not be aroused by their partner. Depression and stress also contribute to poor arousal. The presence of morning erections distinguishes psychological from organic impotence.

EVALUATION OF IMPOTENCE

Men who experience erectile dysfunction should have a thorough evaluation by their physician, including a rectal and genital examination. A careful history regarding medical conditions, past surgery, and medication use should be given to the doctor. As part of the evaluation, blood chemistry screening and hormone levels may be checked. Specific details regarding sexual dysfunction should be discussed. It is important to note the duration and type of problem as well as whether morning erections are still present. Stress, fatigue, anger, and discord in the home or workplace can add to the problem. Most of the time, an accurate diagnosis can be reached from the detailed history and physical examination, but occasionally further testing will be necessary. Mostly, these various tests assess blood flow in the penis. At times, nighttime monitoring is done to determine if erections occur. Erections during dreaming are normal; if there are none, it could indicate that the nerve or blood supply to the penis is not adequate for erection.

SEXUAL DYSFUNCTION IN PARKINSON'S DISEASE

Decreased frequency of sexual behavior has been noted in some Parkinson's disease patients. This may be due to a lessening of libido, which is reported for both partners, or decreased opportunity because of altered motor control. Some spouses relate a change in the level of attraction they feel for their affected partner, and this can contribute to withdrawal from sexual contact. Other uncontrollable symptoms that may make intimacy difficult are an expressionless face, involuntary movements, excess drooling or poor bladder control. Many couples sleep apart because of the nighttime movement disorder, further decreasing the likelihood of physical contact. Lastly, spouses may find it difficult to switch from the caregiving role to a more sensual one.

In particular, women with Parkinson's disease are more likely to have a loss of libido and avoidance of sex than their male counterparts. They report low self-esteem and a loss of sex appeal. Women may also describe more difficulty getting aroused and a change in the ability to have an orgasm. Vaginal dryness as well as muscular rigidity can lead to painful intercourse. Estrogen creams or vaginal lubricants are sometimes used to ease dryness.

Men with Parkinson's disease are more likely to report a decreased ability to achieve and maintain erection. Many will relate a high rate of unsuccessful intercourse. In certain cases, a lack of nocturnal erections points to an organic rather than a psychological cause. The exact mechanism behind the failure of erection in men with Parkinson's disease is not known but probably stems from a combination of physical and mental factors. Medications typically used to treat Parkinson's disease do not cause impotence. There have been rare reports of impotence associated with use of an older dopamine agonist, bromocriptine (Parlodel). Of interest historically, levodopa was felt to act as an aphrodisiac and we do see cases of hypersexuality from levodopa treatment. This excessive sexual expression usually responds to lowering the dosage of medication. Patients who are impotent will not reverse this problem with use of levodopa, even though that treatment may improve their motor ability.

TREATMENT OPTIONS FOR NONORGANIC IMPOTENCE

Addressing underlying psychological factors is the key to treatment of nonorganic impotency. Counseling with a psychotherapist or a sex counselor can help a couple to experience a closer, more loving relationship. This process encourages open discussion of specific fears and desires. However, some people choose to bypass the psychological roots of the problem and treat impotency with medications to induce erection (refer to the treatment section for organic impotency below).

TREATMENT OPTIONS FOR ORGANIC IMPOTENCY

First, there must be optimal management of medical illness or hormonal deficiency. This usually does not improve impotency but will slow further worsening. Treat drug or alcohol dependency, if present. Your physician can change possible offending medications to others with fewer side effects.

Several new medications exist for impotency. They differ in their routes of administration and in their effectiveness. Medications taken by mouth include yohimbine (Yocon) and sildenafil (Viagra). Yohimbine blocks constriction of blood vessels, allowing blood to flow into the penis more readily. It must be taken three times a day regardless of sexual activity. Shown to be about 20 to 30 percent effective, it is primarily used for psychogenic impotence. Yohimbine cannot be used with certain antidepressants and antipsychotics. Sildenafil (Viagra) is the newest agent available for impotence. Its record sales and media coverage have brought about a heightened awareness of the problem faced by millions of men. This agent is effective for organic, mixed, and nonorganic impotency. Sexual stimulation leads to a cascade of reactions that ultimately relaxes the muscles of the penis, allowing the inflow of blood and erection. Viagra inhibits an enzyme that works against this process, thus increasing the likelihood of erection by three to four times, though there is no effect of the pill without sexual stimulation. Viagra should be taken 30 minutes to four hours prior to intercourse. It is an excellent choice for couples who are infertile because of male impotence as it does not affect the sperm. The cost is approximately ten dollars per pill. The most common side effects are headache, flushing, and gastric upset. Viagra should never be used in combination with nitrates as this may lower blood pressure. Table 2 lists some commonly prescribed nitrates. As always, check with your doctor regarding other possible drug interactions.

The injectable medications used for impotence are papaverine and alprostadil (Caverject). Papaverine is used to relax smooth muscle, particularly in large arteries. It is contraindicated in those with heart conduction problems and is not FDA-approved for use in impotency. Injectable alprostadil (Caverject) is a safe and effective way to obtain a natural erection. The active ingredient is prostaglandin E_1, a naturally occurring lipid. Prostaglandin E_1 serves to relax smooth muscle, allowing the spaces in the penis to fill with blood. Erection occurs 5 to 15 minutes after injecting the medication and lasts about 45 minutes. There is a very small risk of sustained erection, lasting more than four hours, and scarring of tissue.

A new delivery system for alprostadil named Muse has been developed. It is now possible to insert the medication into the end of the penis using an applicator. There are four dosage strengths of Muse available. Men should urinate prior to using this medication. Onset of effect is within 5 to 10 minutes and erection lasts 30 to 60 minutes. Those with Parkinson's disease who have tremor or decreased motor control may find this method easier than injection. The primary side effect is possible pain in the penis. Lowered blood pressure or sustained erection may also occur. Female partners have complained of vaginal itching from the medication. It is not recommended to use Muse with a female who is pregnant or of childbearing potential unless a condom is also used.

The mechanical devices that aid in erection are vacuum devices and prosthetic penile implants. A vacuum device draws blood into the penis through vacuum pressure. Placing a band at the base of the penis then

TABLE 2
COMMONLY PRESCRIBED NITRATES,
BY CLASS

- Nitroglycerin
  - —Deponit
  - —Minitran
  - —Nitrek
  - —Nitro-bid
  - —Nitrodisc
  - —Nitro-Dur
  - —Nitrogard
  - —Nitroglyn
  - —Nitrolingual spray
  - —Nitrol ointment
  - —Nitrong
  - —Nitro-Par
  - —Nitrostat
  - —Nitro-Time
  - —Transderm-Nitro

- Isosorbide Mononitrate
  - —Imdur
  - —Ismo
  - —Monoket tablets

- Isosorbide Dinitrate
  - —Dilatrate-SR
  - —Isordil
  - —Sorbitrate

- Erythatyl Tetranitrate

- Pentaerythritol Tetranitrate

- Sodium Nitroprusside

traps the blood. A good device can be costly, but frequent users will find it cost-effective over time. Problems that some men experience with the vacuum device are loss of spontaneity, difficulty ejaculating, and poor blood circulation in the penis after prolonged banding. Penile prosthetic devices provide a permanent solution to impotence. There are two types, semi-rigid rods or inflatable cylinders, which can be implanted inside the penis; safety and efficacy are about the same between the two types. This method is irreversible because the erectile tissue is disrupted. Following the procedure, all erections require the device. Possible adverse events are infection after the procedure, erosion of the device through the penis, and malfunction of the device (primarily the inflatable type).

CONCLUSION

Impotence, although commonly experienced in the aging male population, is more likely to occur in males with Parkinson's disease, especially as the disease advances. Those who experience impotence should have a thorough evaluation by their physician. If there is interest in pursuing a more active sex life, new treatments are available, but the type of treatment depends on the underlying cause of sexual dysfunction. Generally, improved management of Parkinson's disease does not improve sexual function. Medications used to treat Parkinson's disease usually do not bring about impotence, so other causes need to be considered. Occasionally, hypersexuality may be experienced while taking these drugs and may respond to lowering the doses. Women with Parkinson's disease are encouraged to talk about their sexuality so that we will have a better understanding and start to develop ways to help them. For those with vaginal dryness, vaginal lubricants or estrogen creams can be used. Women who experience accidental loss of urine during sexual activity need to speak with their doctor. Couples should learn to communicate about expectations, fears, and desires to avoid misunderstandings and alienation. This will help them to maintain closeness and intimacy even if the sexual act cannot be completed.

In summary, there are three important points to remember. First, be spontaneous in order to take advantage of periods of good motor ability. Second, accept new roles in the relationship to ease tension, and allow for new roles during sex to accommodate physical impairments. Finally, explore avenues for intimacy that do not rely on physical performance but are satisfying to you both.

FOR MORE INFORMATION
ABOUT IMPOTENCE

American Foundation for Urological Disease, Inc.
1-800-242-2383

Impotence World Association/ Impotence Anonymous
1-800-669-1603

The Sexuality Information and Education Council of the United States
    (SIECUS)
130 West 42nd Street, Suite 350
New York, NY 10036
1-212-819-9770

9

Speech, Swallowing, and Communication

Janet Schwantz

Communication—the ability to make our needs known, to express our desires, hopes, and dreams—is an important part of our lives. We use communication in some form every hour of every day. Remember what it is like to have laryngitis or to be in the presence of a group of people who are speaking another language. The person who can't communicate feels left out and excluded from life at these times.

Recent research has indicated that approximately 75 percent of people with Parkinson's disease exhibit changes in their speech and communication as their disease progresses. As with other areas of Parkinson's disease, changes in speech vary from person to person. Because communication is so vital to quality of life, it is important that people with Parkinson's disease and their families understand the possible changes that may occur and act in a timely fashion to accommodate them.

The changes of speech typically occur in a gradual manner, with the parkinsonian patient and family members becoming accustomed to the changes, even to the point of accepting them as normal. Many times the person with Parkinson's disease or a family member will report that the patient has always been soft-spoken. The parkinsonian may believe it is not his or her soft speech that is causing the problem, but that the listener is hard of hearing. We have a saying at our clinic that it is "the law" that a person who has Parkinson's disease must have a spouse who is hard of hearing. This, of course, is not true, but any hearing loss should be dealt with in both the parkinsonian and the family members.

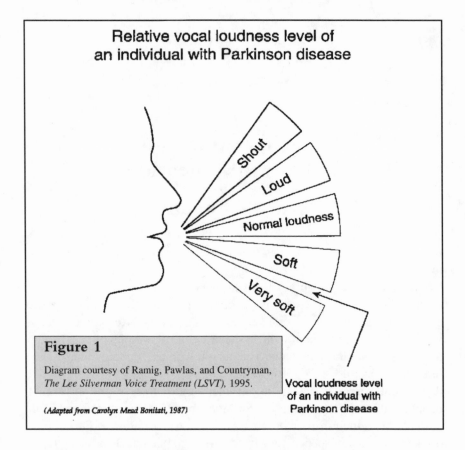

Relative vocal loudness level of an individual with Parkinson disease

Shout
Loud
Normal loudness
Soft
Very soft

Figure 1

Diagram courtesy of Ramig, Pawlas, and Countryman, *The Lee Silverman Voice Treatment (LSVT)*, 1995.

(Adapted from Carolyn Mead Bonitati, 1987)

Vocal loudness level of an individual with Parkinson disease

SPEECH CHARACTERISTICS

Many changes in the speech of a person with Parkinson's disease may occur during the course of the disease. The parkinsonian may experience one or more of the following characteristics:

1. *Low volume or quiet voice (see figure 1).* This is the most commonly reported change in speech. If the parkinsonian has to repeat 25 percent of what he or she says or if the listeners seem to be straining to hear, the loudness level of speech is too low for comfortable conversation. If the person with Parkinson's disease is required to repeat the message very often, any of several consequences may occur. The need for frequent repetitions may lead to frustration for both speaker and listener and tempers may flare, or the person with Parkinson's disease will give up and withdraw from the conversation or social encounter.

2. *Fading voice.* A fading voice is exhibited when the speaker uses a good loudness level at the beginning of the sentence but the voice

becomes quieter by the the end of the sentence, often to the point of a whisper. Fading can also occur for individual words. The last syllable or sound becomes so quiet that it cannot be heard. This reduction in loudness—fading—can affect the listener's understanding of what is said. For example, there is a big difference between the words "bag" and "bat," but if the voice fades and the last sound cannot be heard, the message will be unclear and will require repetition.

3. *Monotone voice.* Changing pitch or using inflection in the voice gives meaning to sentences. A rising pitch at the end of a sentence makes it a question and may change the meaning of the sentence. The following sentences have very different meanings depending on the pitch or inflection, although the words are exactly the same : "He called on Friday." "He called on Friday?" The inability to use inflection in a sentence can lead to misunderstanding and frustration. A monotone voice can also lead the listener to believe the speaker is depressed, mad, or uninterested because the voice sounds so flat. Misunderstandings can arise.

4. *Breathy, tremulous, or hoarse voice.* The Parkinson's disease patient may sound as if he or she has a cold or laryngitis, although the throat is not sore nor does he or she have a cold. This can be compounded by the feeling of drainage or phlegm in the throat. It is often difficult to listen to someone who sounds as if it is hurting him/her to talk. Family members may request that the Parkinson's disease patient "rest" his or her voice, mistakenly thinking that talking is painful. This situation reduces conversation.

5. *Indistinct pronunciation.* Family members and friends may report that the speech of the person with Parkinson's disease sounds "mushy" or "garbled" and difficult to understand. The parkinsonian does not know what to do to "fix" his or her speech in this situation.

6. *Uncontrolled repetition.* Uncontrolled repetition is described as similar to stuttering but different in that the speech gets faster and faster as the Parkinson's disease patient continues to speak. As the conversation continues, the person with Parkinson's disease becomes even more difficult to understand, resulting in frustration for both the parkinsonian and the listener.

The person with Parkinson's disease may exhibit only one or two of the characteristics described. Untreated, the parkinsonian's speech may demonstrate a number of these characteristics. Mild changes occur in speech even in the earliest stages of the disease and should be dealt with at that time, so that more severe problems may be delayed or even prevented. It is important for the person with Parkinson's disease or a family member to ask the physician for a referral to a speech/language pathologist when the first signs of speech changes occur in order to identify speech difficulties and develop treatment strategies.

THE MECHANICS OF SPEECH

Speech is a complex activity using many muscles in specific order to complete making even one simple utterance. Because the person with Parkinson's disease has been speaking for so many years, it is difficult to realize the complex steps involved. Changes in speech may occur in three separate areas: respiration, phonation, and articulation.

Resipiration

Respiration refers to breath support and the act of taking air in (inhalation) and using that air to produce speech as the air goes out of the lungs (exhalation). The muscle rigidity common in the legs and arms of people with Parkinson's disease is also present in the muscles of the lungs and diaphragm. This rigidity may make filling the lungs with air when inhaling and controlling the release of air when speaking during exhalation difficult. This difficulty may result in short rushes of speech or beginning a sentence but running out of air before reaching its end. Either way, the listener will miss part of the message.

Phonation

Phonation refers to the activity of the vocal cords (or vocal folds) which are located in the larynx (often referred to as the "voice box"). The vocal cords are muscles which can stretch easily and vibrate to create the sounds used to produce speech. Because of the muscle rigidity in the vocal cords of people with Parkinson's disease, the vocal cords are stretched, lose some of their elasticity, and become "bowed." Think of the vocal cords as a rubber band. When a rubber band is stretched out for a long time, it loses its elasticity. When the rubber band is released, it is "floppy" and does not return to its original shape. Similarly, the vocal cords of people with Parkinson's disease stretch and lose their elasticity. This loss of elasticity keeps the vocal cords from vibrating as fast or coming together tightly. This inability of the vocal cords to close completely allows too much air to escape and results in reduced loudness or a quiet voice. The movement of the vocal cords also gives the voice "life" by changing pitch and inflection. These changes can make the voice monotone, giving the impression of disinterest, sadness, or depression. The loss of elasticity of the vocal cords happens over an extended period of time and the resulting changes often go unnoticed by the person with Parkinson's disease. Family members and friends begin to have difficulty hearing or understanding the person with Parkinson's disease and may frequently ask for repetition. The person with Parkinson's disease may become frustrated and give up trying to be heard.

Articulation

The third area of speech involves the muscles of the face, lips, tongue, and jaw, all of which allow for clear and precise articulation. When rigidity occurs in these muscles, the speech may sound "slurred" or it may sound like the person is mumbling. The muscle rigidity does not cause weakness but results in reduced ability to move these facial muscles.

SPEECH EVALUATION

A speech evaluation must be completed by a certified speech/language pathologist (SLP), and a referral from the physician for the evaluation is required. A speech/language pathologist is a health care professional trained to evaluate and treat individuals with speech, language, and swallowing problems. The SLP has earned a graduate degree and must be certified by the American Speech-Language and Hearing Association. The speech evaluation may last from 60 to 90 minutes and is a painless procedure. The SLP will evaluate the speed and ease of movement of the jaw, lips, and tongue. Measurements will be taken of loudness levels during several different speech tasks and the Parkinson's disease patient will be tested for his/her ability to control the voice. Trial therapy tasks will be conducted to determine if the person with Parkinson's disease can make changes in his/her voice similar to tasks required in speech therapy sessions. The SLP will discuss the findings of the evaluation with the person with Parkinson's disease and family members and will make recommendations for the goals of therapy to fit the specific speech problem areas identified.

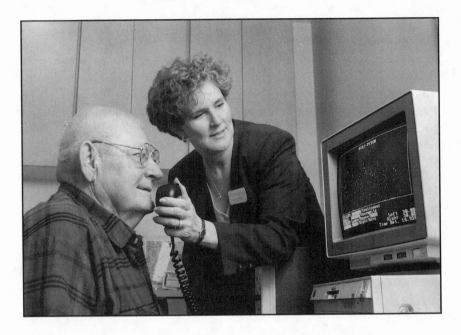

SPEECH THERAPY

Speech therapy can be conducted in many different settings but must be given by a certified SLP with a physician referral. SLPs work in hospitals, rehabilitation centers, and private clinics, which gives the patient many options to choose from. Speech therapy is most successful if the SLP has experience working with the speech changes associated with Parkinson's disease. The person with Parkinson's disease should feel comfortable asking the SLP about his/her amount of experience.

The speech therapy that has been proven to be most successful for Parkinson's disease is called the *Lee Silverman Voice Treatment*. This method focuses on increasing loudness. The act of increasing loudness has the added benefit of increasing breath support, slowing speech down, and improving pronunciation. The SLP will show the person with Parkinson's disease how to achieve and maintain an appropriate level of loudness during the therapy sessions and provide homework assignments to be practiced at home.

Many people with Parkinson's disease request facial exercises to reduce the rigidity of muscles in the face and jaw. It may be helpful to begin with stretching exercises for the face, such as alternating smiling and then puckering the lips or opening the mouth as wide as possible, holding for a count of 5 and then relaxing. A few repetitions of each exercise may relax the facial muscles to prepare for the other speech practice exercises assigned by the SLP.

The benefits of speech therapy include increased loudness, increased vocal quality (reduction of hoarseness and breathiness), increased phonatory stability (reduction of tremor with breath support), and increased overall intelligibility of speech. If the patient has had Parkinson's disease for many years and speech therapy does not completely restore effective communication, amplification devices are used to enhance the loudness of the voice. The appropriate device for the individual patient must be chosen carefully with the help and recommendations of the SLP.

It is important that Parkinson's disease patients be evaluated and treated with speech therapy when speech is only mildly affected. The greatest progress can be made at that time. If the person with Parkinson's disease waits until his or her speech is severely affected, it will be very difficult to make changes in voice and the therapy will not be as successful. Early intervention is the key. The person with Parkinson's disease must be willing to practice his or her speech exercises every day, just as he/she must take the Parkinson's disease medicine every day, in order to maintain good speech and to be able to communicate in all family and social situations.

GENERAL SUGGESTIONS FOR IMPROVING COMMUNICATION

It is important that the person with Parkinson's disease and the listener work together to improve the communication environment. There are several steps that can be taken to aid the Parkinson's disease patient and the listener in keeping the lines of communication open. These include:

For the Person with Parkison's Disease:

• Keep in mind that your ability to speak clearly now requires your conscious and deliberate effort and attention.

• Take a breath before you start to speak and pause between sentences or phrases.

- Encourage your family and friends to ask you to speak louder. This is helpful if you improve when reminded and have no objection to being told.

- Finish saying the final consonant of a word before starting to say the next word. Precise word endings are necessary to differentiate word meanings.

- Express your ideas in short, concise phrases or sentences. Long, involved sentences are often impossible for your listener to comprehend.

- Take your time in organizing your thoughts and try to plan what you are going to say. If you are having trouble thinking of a specific word to express an idea (this may occur particularly in anxious situations), try to think of an associated word to get your idea across.

- Face your listener. It will be easier for you and your listener to communicate if you are facing each other and have each other's full attention.

- Talk for yourself. Don't get into the habit of letting others do all the talking for you.

For Family and Friends:

- Give the person with Parkinson's disease your full and complete attention. Make sure you face each other so that you can watch the patient's mouth for cues as to the word he/she is saying.

- Prompt the person with Parkinson's disease to speak louder. Stand at a distance from him/her and tell him/her to imagine you are in the next room and that he/she needs to "shout" in order for you to hear.

- If the person with Parkinson's disease has problems initiating speech, allow him or her ample time to get started without interrupting his/her concentration.

- Ask the person with Parkinson's disease to rephrase his/her message. His/her alternate choice of words may be more easily understood.

- Give the person with Parkinson's disease feedback, such as an affirmative headshake or "yes" to indicate you understand what he or she is saying. Conversely, let him/her know if you do not understand. Repeat what you did understand and ask him/her to continue from there.

- Ask the person with Parkinson's disease to spell words you cannot understand. Repeat each letter.

- If the person with Parkinson's disease can write legibly, encourage him/her to use writing as a supplement to speech.

- In those cases where speech is severely impaired and generally unintelligible and writing is illegible, an alternative means of communication should be considered.

SWALLOWING

Approximately 50 percent of people with Parkinson's disease notice changes or difficulty with chewing, eating, or swallowing. Changes in swallowing can occur at any stage of Parkinson's disease and range from mild to moderate. Swallowing is a complicated set of muscle movements. Because swallowing is viewed as an automatic reflex, people frequently think that no control can be exerted when something goes wrong. This is not true. Changes in swallowing can be made during eating which will continue to make it a safe and pleasurable experience as well as ensuring good nutrition.

There are several indicators of possible swallowing problems which include:

- Coughing or "strangling" while eating or drinking.

- "Wet" sound in the voice following eating or drinking.

- Throat clearing when eating or drinking.

- Increased effort to eat or drink.

- Increased length of time required to eat a meal.

- Weight loss or dehydration.

- Fever or pneumonia.

Swallowing problems are experienced at three different stages: in the mouth, in the throat, and in the esophagus. Chewing the food and moving it out of the mouth is the first step involved in swallowing. The textures of food are important and should be considered carefully. The food must be chewed and moved through the mouth in a cohesive form and then the tongue must drop down in the back to allow the food to go into the throat. Problems can occur with this process if the liquid or food travels too fast or is not chewed adequately and enters the throat in a noncohesive form or ball. Because of the muscle rigidity found in Parkinson's disease, the tongue will not drop down to let the food pass into the throat. When this happens, the food falls forward again and the Parkinson's disease patient must chew until the tongue responds appropriately.

The second area of swallowing is in the throat or pharynx. There are several places in the throat where the food or liquid can collect or pool. Since the muscles of the throat are rigid in Parkinson's disease, all the food may not be swallowed and pooling occurs. Usually just a small amount of food is left behind each time, but after several swallows the quantity builds up and can then fall into the airway, causing coughing or choking. The food build-up can even enter the lungs. Food or liquid in the lungs can lead to pneumonia.

The third area of concern in swallowing is at the opening to the esophagus which leads to the stomach. Sometimes muscle rigidity will keep the esophagus from opening wide enough or at the proper time, resulting in food left in the throat to possibly fall into the airway.

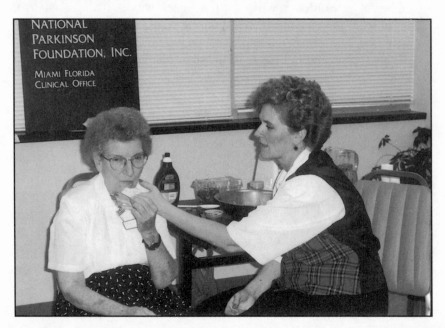

NATIONAL
PARKINSON
FOUNDATION, INC.

MIAMI FLORIDA
CLINICAL OFFICE

HINTS TO AID IN SWALLOWING

Several things can be done to help with swallowing and eating problems. If a person with Parkinson's disease is choking, coughing, or losing weight, he/she should be evaluated by an SLP to identify the problems, advise on best food consistency, and give recommendations for safe positions and schedules for eating. These suggestions might include:

- Before eating, think through the steps of swallowing: lips closed, teeth together, food on tongue—lift tongue up, then back, and swallow (UP-BACK-SWALLOW).

- Eat slowly and in small amounts.

- Take time to chew first on one side of the mouth, then on the other.

- Do not mix liquid and solid food in the mouth at the same time, as the difference in consistency and the rate at which the food passes through the mouth can create problems.

- People with Parkinson's disease should usually not eat food which does not stay together (scatters) in the mouth, such as peas, rice, and corn, unless eaten in a gravy.

Most foods can be eaten by anyone with Parkinson's disease, but the food must be prepared in a safe form or consistency. A caregiver or family member should learn the Heimlich maneuver in case of choking. No two people are alike, so an individualized swallowing program is imperative to safe swallowing.

MEMORY

Memory and cognitive changes may appear at any stage in the progression of Parkinson's disease, but are more often reported by individuals who have had the disease for many years. These changes can interfere with the person's ability to communicate effectively with others. In those individuals who experience cognitive changes, the individual may experience one or more of the following:

- Reduced ability to concentrate or "think through" an activity.

- Additional time required to think of what one wants to say.

- Difficulty thinking of a specific word one wants to use.

- Loss of one's train of thought while speaking.

- Being easily distracted.

- Increased time required to process information.

A certified SLP has extensive training in recognizing and assessing changes that affect the use of language and memory. The SLP also knows strategies and therapy procedures to address memory and cognitive deficits and can recommend recall strategies to aid in carrying out everyday activities. An SLP may be able to help a patient regain more control over planning and preparing for daily routines and events, which can lead to greater independence and self-confidence.

There are many things that the person with Parkinson's disease can do to stimulate "brain power" and improve memory. These include:

- Read and discuss articles in the newspaper.

- Do crossword or "seek and find" puzzles.

- Do flowerpot gardening.

- Become a bird watcher.

- Go through old photos and make memory books for grandchildren.

- Plan a household chore to do every day.

- Keep a detailed diary of daily events.

- Keep paper and pen handy to jot down information to be remembered.

- Organize items on lists by category.

- Focus on remembering main points, not trying to recall every detail.

- Keep a calendar of appointments and engagements to review daily.

Family and friends of people with Parkinson's disease can utilize the following hints to ease communication when memory and concentration changes interfere with daily activities:

- Allow individuals with Parkinson's disease ample time to process what has been said and to respond.

- Be concise when speaking of specific people and events—use proper names rather than pronouns (for example, use "Sally" instead of "she").

- Offer limited choices. For example, when choosing food for dinner, say, "Would you like chicken or beef?" rather than, "What would you like for dinner?"

- Review activities for the day every morning.

- Perform activities of daily living in the same order every day. People who have memory problems function better during the day if they know what is going to happen and when.

While many people with Parkinson's disease never develop memory and cognitive changes, the recommendations presented here can help individuals who do experience difficulties in this area to better cope with and compensate for the changes and enhance functional levels and self-esteem.

CONCLUSION

Communication impacts every area of life every day. The reduction of communication ability or the loss of communication creates a great strain on the quality of life. It is important to recognize the possible changes in communication ability and swallowing function caused by Parkinson's disease. Education is important, and early intervention through evaluation and speech/swallowing therapy is the key. Changes in speech or memory should be reported to the physician immediately. Don't wait!! It is much easier to learn effective strategies and techniques to keep the speech mechanism functional than it is to rebuild what may have been lost.

REFERENCES

Ramig, L., Pawlas, A., and Countryman, S. (1995). *The Lee Silverman Voice Treatment (LSVT): A Practical Guide to Treating the Voice and Speech Disorders in Parkinson Disease.* Iowa City: University of Iowa, National Center for Voice and Speech. Phone: 1-319-335-6602.

10

Causes and Prevention of Falls in Parkinson's Disease

Jeffrey W. Elias and Trudy Hutton

THE FACTS ABOUT FALLS IN PARKINSON'S DISEASE AND NORMAL AGING

For people over the age of 65, falling is the most common accident leading to an injury and as such represents a major health risk. Statistically, it is expected that one-fourth to one-third of individuals over age 65 will fall during a year's time and half of these people will fall more than once. Twenty-five percent of these falls would be expected to require medical attention. Minor injuries are more common than serious injuries, but 5 percent of "fallers" will receive a serious soft-tissue injury. Another 5 percent will suffer a bone fracture or require hospitalization, with 1 percent of these sustaining a hip fracture. Wrist and hip fractures account for 25 percent of total bone fractures. Although only 1 percent of falls result in a hip fracture, a femur/hip fracture produces one of the longest hospital stays and is one of the most serious consequences of a fall. Hip fractures are also expensive and account for about 70 percent of the estimated total cost of 1.5 million fractures per year in the elderly.

Both increased age and female gender make an individual more susceptible to a fall. As might be expected, older people are more likely to suffer a serious injury from a fall. The ratio of falls to fractures increases from 200 to 1 to 10 to 1 from age 65 to 85. The greater risk of falling for women than men has been attributed to a number of different factors. These factors include differences in lower body strength, more older

144

women, greater longevity, reduced bone mass, menopause-related osteoporosis, and weaker overall muscle strength. These factors also place women at about an 80 percent greater risk for a femur/hip fracture than men. In the United States, the risk for a femur fracture in white women doubles every six or seven years beginning at age 45 and peaking at age 85. For men, the increased risk of femur fracture begins at about age 55, also doubling every six to seven years and peaking at age 85. The risk for femur fracture for men remains about half that of women.

There is rarely one single cause for a fall. Many falls are the result of a combination of environmental factors and individual risk factors. Age, gender, and health and general physical condition are primary vulnerability factors, but not causes of falls. Most falls are the result of several contributing factors including:

- Environmental hazards
- Gait/balance problems
- Muscle weakness
- Poor vision
- Inattention
- Bad judgment.

While vigorous individuals are less likely to fall, the vigor of an activity can influence the nature of injury. Falls that occur during walking are likely to result in an injury to the wrist or hand. Falls that occur while standing or transferring weight typically result in sideward or backward falls and an increased risk of hip fracture. Hip fractures are estimated to be eight times more likely to occur when *turning* than when walking straight.

After a fall, an individual is typically more cautious. In some cases, however, a fear of falling develops that can contribute to future falls due to reluctance to perform the physical actions necessary to maintain posture or strong gait (see figure 1). One large national study reported that 30 percent of individuals who experienced a fall retained a residual fear that interfered with their desire for activity. A single fall can lead to a downward spiral that results in reduced activity and subsequent reduced social and mental stimulation.

There are no statistics on falling available specifically for Parkinson's disease patients, but problems with muscle control, gait, balance, and posture place these patients at increased risk for a fall. Lesser known but significant risk factors for falls in Parkinson's disease patients include changes in vision, eye movements, and control of attention.

Figure 1

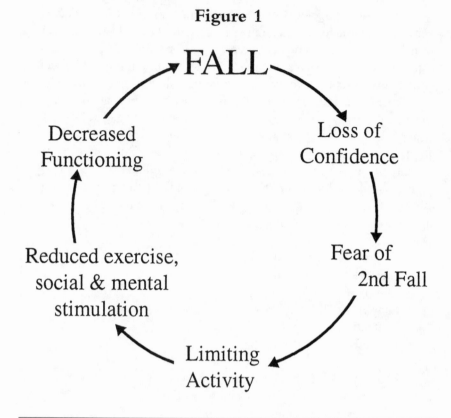

VISION AS A RISK FACTOR FOR FALLS IN PARKINSON'S DISEASE PATIENTS

Changes in vision, many noticeable by middle age, are an inevitable part of the aging process. The basic changes one can expect with age include:

- Reduced acuity and ability to accommodate to changing lighting
- Reduced contrast sensitivity
- Greater sensitivity to glare
- Poorer and slower adaptation to night vision
- Decreased color vision for the blue end of the color spectrum
- Narrowed field of vision, particularly under stress.

Many of the normal changes in vision that occur with aging are the result of structural changes in the lens of the eye. As one grows older, the lens loses the ability to bulge and stretch to accommodate near and far vision. Decreased accommodation (near and far vision focus) can be expected to appear by age 40 to 45, and little accommodation is available with the lens after age 50. After age 50, accommodation is made by moving the head forward and backward or by peering through an artificial lens.

For Parkinson's disease patients, poor control over eye movements adds to the normal age-related changes in vision. As a result, Parkinson's disease patients will encounter difficulty following moving objects with their eyes in a smooth fashion. Almost all Parkinson's disease patients develop a reduced ability to look up ("upgaze") or to look down ("downgaze"). Research finds that 90 percent of Parkinson's disease patients have reduced upgaze and downgaze compared to 10 percent of normal elderly. Consequently, looking up or down results in a greater movement of the head than would normally be expected. Balance and posture tend to follow the position of the head. Moving the head to look upward instead of using only the eyes results in a shift of the head backward and a change in the center of gravity. For Parkinson's disease patients who have a stooped posture, looking upward becomes even more of a challenge and requires greater control to maintain center of gravity and balance. A reduced downgaze in combination with a stooped posture results in increased body sway when looking downward. Many Parkinson's disease patients in the advanced stages of the disease report that when they bend over to look down they lose control of balance.

To reduce risk for the elderly, and especially Parkinson's disease patients, it is wise to change the environment to reduce the need to look up or down. If one is experiencing balance problems or falling, Parkinson's disease patients should not hesitate to ask others to do the reaching down or up for them. Objects that are used routinely should be moved within the "visual-gaze comfort-zone." Recognition of the increased risk for a fall when looking up or down is also important. Looking up and down is reflexive and simple, which makes being cautious difficult. A special warning for the Parkinson's disease patient to avoid the use of chairs or ladders may seem silly, but lifelong habits of independence and climbing are hard to break. It is not just fear that creates greater body sway on chairs and ladders. Just as tall buildings sway more than short buildings, climbing onto a chair will increase the degree of body sway relative to the ground. Moving the head forward or backward to adjust for poor lens accommodation or reduced upgaze increases postural sway even more when standing on an elevated surface. Parkinson's disease patients have a decreased ability to recover from postural instability, and the increased instability created by standing on an elevated surface results in a particularly dangerous situation.

Reduced lens transparency is another change in vision, noticeable about middle age, that results in poor clarity of vision and increased sensitivity to glare. Wearing sunglasses that block both the ultraviolet and blue spectrum of vision helps to reduce the formation of cataracts and damage to the retina, as well as cuts down on glare. Unfortunately, wearing sunglasses can also reduce the amount of light reaching the eye. As we age, the size of the pupil opening is reduced, resulting in less light reaching the eye. In normal daylight conditions, the amount of light reaching the eye at age 60 is one-third of the amount of light reaching the eye at age 20. In low light conditions (dimly lit buildings, at night), that ratio decreases to one-tenth. The combination of reduced pupil opening and the shaded lens of sunglasses can reduce overall vision substantially. Therefore, careful thought should be given to when and where sunglasses are worn. Sunglasses should be put on after going outside, and should be taken off before going inside. Frequently taking off and putting on sunglasses to accommodate to changing light conditions can be a difficult habit to master, but many trips and slips occur entering and exiting areas of changing luminance (e.g., going from a dimly lit building into bright sunlight). Often the risk of a fall can be offset by developing good habits.

Parkinson's disease results in an inherent loss of ability to perceive contrast. This aspect of vision change is particularly frustrating to Parkinson's disease patients because it reduces the ability to clearly see the details of objects and surfaces. *Contrast* refers to the difference in brightness between adjacent areas of a visual stimulus. Objects are seen more easily when there is a distinct difference in brightness between background and object (e.g., writing with dark ink on white paper maximizes contrast). Providing more luminance on objects increases the degree of contrast. The ability to see contrast extends over a range of spatial frequencies, much like a TV tuner permits access to a number of different channels. The perception of dark letters on a white background requires the ability to see high spatial frequency information. High frequency means more visual information per visual angle. For example, an oil painting viewed from close range appears to be nothing but blobs of color. At a close distance, the painting is viewed at a wide visual angle and via the use of low frequency channels (see figure 2). When one steps back from the painting, visual angle is reduced and objects are seen at a higher visual frequency and become recognizable (see figure 3).

Adjustment for contrast is yet another reason the head bobs back and forth when trying to focus on an object or reading material. The high frequency channels of the visual system are particularly important to the ability to detect edges and boundaries between objects.

Low contrast vision is important to see the subtleties of the world.

Figure 2. Wide visual angle: perception is via low frequency channels.

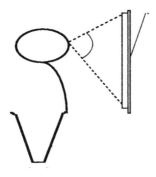

Recognition of faces, subtle features of objects, and the perception of the speed of moving objects all depend upon the ability of the visual system to respond to low frequency visual information. Perception of the speed of one's own movement also depends on the use of the low frequency channels. In addition to reducing the perception of surface characteristics of objects, low light conditions reduce contrast. Visual displays that are low contrast under high luminance conditions become even lower contrast under low luminance conditions. What is viewed at 20/20 vision under high luminance conditions may be viewed at 20/60 vision under low luminance conditions; consequently, one would have to be three times closer to see the same detail under the low luminance condition.

Often we prefer and design low contrast into our environments, even though high contrast is better for detection and recognition of objects. High contrast is energizing, low contrast is soothing. Using low lighting in the evening to establish a warm glow is pleasing, but low lighting can create shadows and reduce contrast. Aesthetics should be kept in balance with safety.

In Parkinson's disease, as well as in normal aging, the loss of contrast sensitivity begins in the high frequency channels and eventually is lost in the low frequency channels. The ability to perceive contrast in visual displays is gradually reduced as Parkinson's disease progresses. Research shows that by stage III of the Hoehn and Yahr scale, significant change in contrast sensitivity can be observed for many patients. Almost all stage IV Parkinson's disease patients experience loss of sensitivity to contrast. The sequence of progression through the Hoehn and Yahr scale is shown below.

Figure 3. Reduced visual angle: perception is via higher frequency channels.

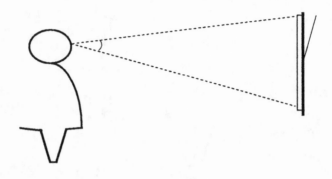

Stage I —symptoms are unilateral, affecting only one side of the body.

Stage II —symptoms are bilateral, but balance is not impaired.

Stage III—symptoms are bilateral and balance is affected; the person remains physically independent.

Stage IV—Parkinson's disease is functionally disabling; the person requires assistance to stand or walk.

Stage V —the patient is confined to a bed or chair.

It is important to note that stage III also signals significant changes in postural stability that may be accentuated by changes in vision. Patients experiencing contrast sensitivity loss frequently express frustration with the failure of eyeglasses to improve vision. Unfortunately, the problem is not one of focus or accommodation. Attempts to increase contrast in the environment or raise luminance levels are useful, but at some point greater luminance does not offset the perceptual loss. The reason for the loss of high frequency sensitivity is unknown, but may be related to a loss of dopamine in the retina. There are, however, relatively few dopaminergic cells in the retina, so it may be an imbalance in neurotransmitters that causes the problem, not just the reduction of dopamine.

The loss of high frequency vision increases the risk for a fall due to the inability to identify edges, corners, or the nature of floor surfaces. In some cases, a decreased ability to plan how high to lift the foot or how far to swing the leg to avoid objects is the result of reduced ability to perceive contrast. When loss of contrast sensitivity becomes apparent, effort needs to be made to improve lighting to make it easier to use the high frequency channels and reduce shadows or glare, and to move furniture whose edges are not easily detected. Uncluttered environments can reduce the number of visual confusions possible. Sometimes attractive floor coverings high in contrast can become confusing and result in an uncertain gait when the contrast in the floor covering cannot be easily detected. This is more likely to occur under low luminance than high luminance conditions.

GAIT, POSTURE, AND FALLS RISK IN PARKINSON'S DISEASE

Walking requires the ability to maintain postural control and dynamic (moving) balance while propelling the body through space with only the feet in contact with a surface. Body weight must be supported and momentum must be initiated, maintained, and controlled via muscular and nervous system mechanisms. The movement mechanism is one of self-propulsion, so balance is consistently lost and equilibrium regained while walking. At some point in the walk cycle, only one foot is on the ground and the body center of gravity moves forward beyond the body until the opposite swinging leg comes forward and the heel strikes the ground. At this point, the cycle begins again. A smooth gait requires anticipation of shifts in balance and coordination of head, eye, trunk, arm, hip, leg, knee, ankle, and foot movements. Adaptation to changes in ground surface, direction, and speed of movement must be made. One must have confidence that this complex task can be accomplished (reduced fear of falling). Postural stability, both standing and walking, requires an integration of visual, proprioceptive (muscles and joints), and vestibular stimulation sensory feedback.

Parkinson's disease negatively affects all of the factors required for a smooth gait: posture, dynamic balance, propulsion, momentum, anticipation of movement, and muscular control. Loss of vestibular function is not well established for Parkinson's disease patients, but patients who find themselves relying primarily on vestibular input for balance are clearly compromised by stage III. For example, standing in a dark movie theater on a sloping surface momentarily places a greater demand on vestibular input for balance because of poor sensory input to the visual and proprioceptive (lower body muscle and joints) senses. Parkinson's disease patients are likely to have more difficulty controlling postural sway (movement around the center of gravity) due to poor sensory integration and inefficient muscle action. Studies of muscle action in Parkinson's disease patients during walking, standing, or sitting frequently find:

1. Muscles tend to work continuously rather than in a cycle.
2. There is a reduced level of muscle activation.
3. Muscles that would normally work in alternate fashion are simultaneously activated and work against each other.

Research shows that there is a clear difference between patients in stage II and stage III with respect to the ability to quickly adapt posture to changing or uneven ground surfaces. Thus, stage III and stage IV patients in particular need to be aware of the difficulty of maintaining posture when standing on sloping or uneven surfaces. While gently sloping ramps may be easier to negotiate than steps, steeply sloping ramps may be difficult.

Gait and posture are judged clinically in Parkinson's disease via a number of different measures. One of the most common measures of gait and ambulation comes from the United Parkinson's Disease Rating Scales (UPDRS). This scale rates patients as:

0 = normal
1 = mild difficulty (may not swing arms or may drag leg)
2 = moderate difficulty (exhibits short steps or difficulty turning, but requires little or no assistance)
3 = severe disturbance of walking (exhibits festination, propulsion, or freezing, necessitating assistance with a walker, cane, etc., at least half the time)
4 = cannot walk at all, even with assistance.

This assessment focuses on the general degree of motion of the arms and legs, length of steps, number of steps, velocity of movement, ability to turn, tendency to freeze, and need for assistance. The greater the alteration of gait, the greater the risk for a fall. This assessment of gait and ambulation measure, although a rather brief scale, is very helpful in predicting risk for falls in Parkinson's disease patients.

Parkinson's disease patients typically walk more slowly, with a variable and reduced step length. As Parkinson's disease progresses, the patient's gait characteristically can be described as stooped in posture and shuffling in pattern. The degree of arm movement is reduced and demonstrates a general appearance of reduced body movement. Due to reduced leg lift and flexibility, the toes may barely clear the walking surface. This is particularly likely when the individual is tired. The reduced degree of body movement reflects the reduced angle of movement for joints. These factors alter the gait and the normal heel-strike-and-roll-forward foot action required to push or propel off one foot while landing on the other.

Parkinson's disease patients have particular difficulty with initiation and control of ongoing momentum. When momentum is uncontrolled, a festinating gait may appear. This gait is characterized by short and rapid steps and the appearance that the individual is propelled forward into almost a running mode. Festination can occur without stooped posture and the balance shifted forward, although the stooped posture and forward weight shift certainly add to the effect.

Sometimes freezing occurs, in which case the individual is unable to initiate momentum. Freezing is the name given to the temporary involuntary inability to move and is fairly common among people with advanced Parkinson's disease. Freezing often occurs when individuals are about to enter a doorway, turn a corner, come upon sudden obstructions, walk in narrow hallways or in crowds, or feel stress to perform. The cause of this extremely frustrating gait disturbance is unknown. Given the difficulty that Parkinson's disease patients have in integrating motor movement and perception, the need to change the movement direction as the impending object, turn, or doorway approaches may interfere with ongoing movement. There is no specific means of getting started again after freezing occurs. Patients often develop unique methods of initiating movement, such as knee rocking or personal verbal initiation. Other suggestions include:

- changing direction
- humming a march beat
- counting out loud (1-2-3, 1-2-3) and moving to the count
- visualizing a successful action
- focusing on a specific object ahead
- pretending to step over objects or cracks.

Inability to perceive or generate a higher rate of optic flow while walking has been suggested to influence freezing, but this is still a point of speculation. Optic flow is generated in peripheral vision as one moves through the environment. Researchers suggest that perception of our own movement speed in peripheral vision provides a means of feedback by which to regulate gait speed. The slowed Parkinson's gait reduces this type of feedback. Even if we are still, objects moving past us provide a feeling of motion: for example, a car moving past us at a stoplight makes us feel like we are moving. A popular computer screensaver that has objects moving from the center to the periphery of the screen at a rapid rate provides a feeling of movement. One Parkinson's disease patient has developed a number of devices to artificially increase the rate of optical flow and reports them to be successful. Some suggestions to increase the perception of optic flow are to place designs at the ends of passageways that will appear to expand outward as you approach them. Concentric squares or circles will produce this effect. Wall designs that accentuate peripheral perception of movement will improve the perception of optical flow as well. Before redecorating the house, however, one should remember the issue of optical flow in gait management is still speculative.

EXECUTIVE FUNCTION AND FALLS IN PARKINSON'S DISEASE PATIENTS

Gait, balance, and vision difficulties are not the only risk factors for falls in Parkinson's disease patients. Cognitive processes play a role as well. The motor symptoms in Parkinson's disease arise from degeneration and imbalance of neurotransmitters in the subcortical–basal ganglia area of the brain. There are reciprocal neural pathways in the brain between the basal ganglia and the frontal lobe. A disruption in the functioning of these pathways results in cognitive symptoms typically related to frontal system decline. In Parkinson's disease, this results in individuals who are typically oriented, aware of surroundings, have understanding of time, and have general knowledge but are cognitively inefficient.

The cognitive inefficiency associated with Parkinson's disease appears early in the disease process and is demonstrated by increased distractibility, inattention, and forgetfulness. In the later stages of the disease, planning and organizing are affected. In addition, the person with more advanced disease demonstrates reduced adaptability to novel situations, failure to accurately monitor his own activities, and apathy. These changes in cognition are referred to as loss of "executive function" or ability to carry out goal-directed behavior. Research shows that by Hoehn and Yahr stage III executive functions begin to show impairment. This makes stage III a watershed for Parkinson's disease patients—that is, balance, vision, and cognition are all more likely to contribute to a fall at this stage. However, increased distractibility and inattentiveness, which are normal cognitive changes expected with increased age, are affected in stage II Parkinson's disease. By stage IV Parkinson's disease, executive functions are clearly impaired. Fatigue, stress, depression, medication, or too much alcohol can affect executive functions in anyone. Such conditions for Parkinson's disease patients can accentuate executive function failure and the risk for a fall. Parkinson's patients are particularly susceptible to "environmental dependency," which refers to a situation in which a stimulus in the environment—particularly a stimulus that triggers a habitual action—takes over ongoing behavior. An example of this behavior would be rushing to answer a ringing doorbell or telephone, hurrying outside in the morning to get the newspaper, or racing to the bathroom. When executive function fails, habitual actions take over behavior. Furniture that is moved out of place and navigated around carefully under conditions of full attention can be completely forgotten under conditions of environmental dependency.

In a familiar and predictable environment, habits and environmental dependency can sometimes actually help a person through the day. In an unfamiliar environment, such as that encountered when visiting another person's home, a hotel, or a hospital, familiar patterns of behavior related to the old environment can result in an accident in the new surroundings. This tendency for Parkinson's disease patients to rely on old routines and behaviors in new situations has to be carefully considered to avoid a fall. For example, waking in the middle of the night and having to find a strange bathroom is a prime situation for old habits and anticipated environmental pathways to take precedence over the new behaviors required. The use of a nightlight in unfamiliar surroundings can help signal the presence of a novel environment upon waking. Similar situations arise when modifications are made to a familiar environment. It is easy to forget that the back steps are being repaired when hurrying to take out the garbage. Signs posted on the back door to remind one of the repairs may be ignored. Preventing easy use of the back door could prevent a nasty fall.

The combination of gait, balance, vision, and cognitive changes in Parkinson's disease makes certain areas of the environment more likely to produce a fall. Research shows that Parkinson's disease patients in stage III and stage IV have increased difficulty in adapting to uneven, soft, or tilted surfaces such as those found outside in grassy areas. Transition areas such as doorways typically require greater attention to gait, vision, balance, and cognition due to potential changes in ground surface (e.g., smooth to rough), elevation, light conditions, or objects to navigate. Transition areas that lie within acceleration areas (routes to the front or back door, bathroom, phone, alarm system) produce a heightened risk due to the typically compelling nature of activities in these areas. Turning areas, particularly those next to furniture, pictures, mail receptacles, or mirrors, can be particularly risky if the activity prior to the turn is likely to be distracting (e.g., looking at one's self in the mirror or reading mail as one enters a doorway). Standing on a throw rug while looking in a bathroom mirror is a likely scenario in many homes. Mirrors and steps are a bad combination, as is talking while walking up or down steps. Carrying objects up or down steps changes the center of gravity forward or backward and makes recovery from a slip or trip practically impossible. Placing objects on a stairway to be moved at a later time with the assumption that they will be avoided is extremely risky.

PERSONAL ADAPTATION
AND FALL PREVENTION

Numerous examples of risk and the means for reducing that risk have been presented. Intrinsic factors such as inattention are hard to combat without some concerted effort to train oneself or a caregiver to be aware of potential risks for falls. Fall prevention requires anticipation and effort. Spotting potential risk situations only requires a heightened awareness. Changing behaviors or living environments requires real dedication. Research with elderly patients shows that building strength and flexibility helps to reduce falls. Similar activities for Parkinson's disease patients can have dramatic effects. Observation in our laboratory shows that apathy in patients often makes them appear to be disinterested in physical exercise, yet when prompted to participate, general well-being is greatly improved.

REFERENCES

Bles, W., and Brandt, T., eds. (1986). *Disorders of Posture and Gait*. Paris: Elsevier.

Cummings, S., et al. (1995). "Risk factors for hip fracture in white women." *New England Journal of Medicine* 332:767–815.

Downton, J. (1998). "Who falls and why?" In M. A. Horan and R. A. Little, eds., *Injury in the Aging*. New York: Cambridge University Press.

Elias, J. W. (1995). "Normal vs. pathological aging: Are we assessing adequately for dementia?" *Experimental Aging Research* 21:97–100.

Elias, J., Hutton, J., Shroyer, T., et al. (1996). "Assessment of falls risk in Parkinsonians." Presented at the International Movement Disorders Congress, Vienna, Austria, 1996.

Elias, J. W., and Treland, J. T. (in press). "Executive function and cognitive rehabilitation in old age." In R. Hill and L. Backman, eds., *Cognitive Rehabilitation in Old Age*. New York: Oxford University Press.

Gibson, M. J., Andres, R.O., Isaacs, B., et al. (1987). "The prevention of falls in later life." *Danish Medical Bulletin* 34 (Supp.) 4:1–24.

Horak, F., Nutt, J., and Nashner, L. (1992). "Postural inflexibility in Parkinsonian subjects." *Journal of the Neurological Sciences* 12: 1–13.

Hughes, P., and Neer, R. (1981). "Lighting for the elderly." *Human Factors* 23:65–85.

Hutton, J., Morris, J., Elias, J., Varma, R., and Poston, J. (1991). "Spatial contrast is reduced in bilateral Parkinson's disease." *Neurology* 41: 1200–1202.

Hutton, J., Shapiro, I., and Christians, B. (1982). "The functional significance of restricted upgaze." *Archives of Physical Medicine and Rehabilitation* 63:617–19.

Jankovich, J., and Tolosa, E., eds. (1988). *Parkinson's Disease and Movement Disorders*, Second Edition. Baltimore: Urban and Schwartzenberg.

Koretz, J., and Handelman, G. (1998). "How the human eye focuses." In *Science's Vision: The Mechanics of Sight*. New York: Scientific American.

Vellas, B., Wayne, S., Garry, P., and Baumgartner, R. (1998). "A two-year longitudinal study of falls in 482 community dwelling elderly adults." *Journals of Gerontology: Medical Science* 53A:M264-M274.

Woollacott, M., Shumway-Cook, A., and Nashner, L. (1986). "Aging and postural control: Changes in sensory organization and muscular coordination." *International Journal of Aging and Human Development* 23:97–114.

Youdim, M., and Riederer, P. (1997). "Understanding Parkinson's disease." *Scientific American* 52:52–59.

11

Ways to Reduce the Risk of Falling in the Home Environment

JoAnn Shroyer and Joan Dickinson

INTRODUCTION

For the first time in the history of the United States, our society has shifted from one of youth (i.e., under the age of 65) to one of age (i.e., over the age of 65). By the year 2000, the U.S. population of those 65 years and older will be over 34 million people and will represent 13 percent of the population (American Association of Retired Persons, 1994; Brawley, 1997; Hutton, Elias, Shroyer, and Curry, 1997; Pirkl, 1994). Not only are the numbers of older people growing, but also older people are living longer. Most people will live 30 to 35 years longer than their parents or grandparents. Once an individual reaches the age of 62, he or she can expect to live an additional 25 years. These increases in life expectancy have changed the structure within the older population, and individuals who are 85 years and older are the fastest growing segment among older adults (American Association of Retired Persons, 1994; Brawley, 1997; Hutton et al., 1997; Pirkl, 1994).

The demographic changes cited above present challenges to many professionals in our society. In particular, the interior design and architecture professions are challenged with providing environments that meet the diverse needs of this special population. When interior environments are improperly designed, healthy individuals can usually adapt and maintain activities. The elderly and individuals with Parkinson's disease do not have this inherent flexibility, and design flaws can lead to falls, injury, or death (Shroyer, 1994). Therefore, the purpose of this chapter is to provide design recommendations and suggestions that may reduce the risk of falling and injury for individuals diagnosed with Parkinson's disease.

SYMPTOMS OF PARKINSON'S DISEASE

Typically, the first symptom to be noticed by the afflicted individual is tremor (Creasey and Broe, 1993; Duvoisin and Sage, 1996; Klawans and Topel, 1974; Pearce, 1992). The tremor that affects the person with Parkinson's disease is a resting tremor that disappears when the person moves or is asleep. The tremor is variable and tends to occur in one or both hands or arms and occasionally in the legs (Pearce, 1992). Certain skills such as using a screwdriver, opening doors and drawers, or tying one's shoes become increasingly difficult as the tremor worsens. The pill-rolling tremor (i.e., tremor between the thumb and forefinger) is frequently seen (Duvoisin and Sage, 1996; Klawans and Topel, 1974; Pearce, 1992).

Another common symptom of Parkinson's disease is rigidity (Creasey and Broe, 1993; Duvoisin and Sage, 1996; Pearce, 1992). With rigidity, the muscles are constantly tensed when they should be relaxed. When a person with Parkinson's disease is lying down, for example, a space between his or her neck and the pillow typically exists because the neck muscles are tensed. Rigidity tends to be seen first in the back of the neck and the shoulders (Pearce, 1992). The individual with Parkinson's disease will typically complain of stiffness, soreness, pain, and cramping. Another form of rigidity is cogwheel rigidity, where resistance in the joints has a cogwheel or rachety quality (Pearce, 1992).

Another cardinal symptom that is experienced by individuals with Parkinson's disease is bradykinesia (i.e., slow movement) (Creasey and Broe 1993; Duvoisin and Sage, 1996; Pearce, 1992). Symptoms of bradykinesia include (a) slow movement, (b) lack of automatic movements (e.g., slowing of arms during walking, eye blinking, saliva production due to lack of automatic swallowing, and reduced facial expressions), (c) tiredness, (d) freezing in the middle of a task, (e) the perception that the individual's feet are glued to the floor, (f) the need for great amounts of concentration when completing a task, (g) difficulty in completing more than one task simultaneously, and (h) shuffling gait (Duvoisin and Sage, 1996; Pearce, 1992). These symptoms lead to difficulty in switching directions when walking, mask-like facial appearances, and lack of spontaneous movement. When healthy individuals walk, they swing either arm with the opposite leg and lead with their head, eyes, and shoulders when turning. Individuals with Parkinson's disease cannot move with a natural, synchronized arm-leg swing and fail to lead with their head when turning. As a result, the person with Parkinson's disease manipulates a turn using his or her body as one piece, which is why freezing tends to occur when a turn is attempted (Duvoisin and Sage, 1996).

Unfortunately, the symptoms associated with Parkinson's disease can lead to falls. Tremor of the legs, shuffling gait, freezing, and rigidity cause the individual with Parkinson's disease to have great difficulty maintaining balance and walking (Hutton et al., 1997). When these symptoms are coupled with environmental hazards such as a torn carpet, stairways, inadequate illumination, a high-pile carpet, or high thresholds, the likelihood of falling and injury increases dramatically.

CAUSES OF FALLING

Falling is considered by many researchers to be multifaceted, and as illustrated in Table 1 and in much of the literature, the causes of falls can be divided into two categories: intrinsic factors and extrinsic factors (Lach et al., 1991; Woolley, Czaja, and Drury, 1997). Intrinsic factors include: (a) gait and balance disorders, (b) mobility problems, (c) sensory problems, (d) neural problems, (e) cognitive problems, (f) medication usage, (g) an increase in age, (h) female gender, (i) muscle weakness, (j) drop attacks (i.e., a sudden fall not due to dizziness or unconsciousness), and (k) orthostatic hypotension (Brown, 1995; Craven and Bruno, 1986; Hutton et al., 1997; Josephson, Fabacher, and Rubenstein, 1991; Lach et al., 1991; Nevitt, Cummings, and Hudes, 1991; Perlin, 1992; Salgado, Lord, Packer, and Ehrlich, 1994; Tinetti, 1989; Ulfarsson and Robinson, 1994). Falls may also occur as a result of extrinsic factors or environmental design hazards. Examples cited in the literature include: (a) poor or inadequate lighting, (b) changes in floor surface (e.g., raised thresholds, transitions between floor materials, use of throw rugs, and torn carpets), (c) slippery floors, (d) a lack of grab bars in the bathroom, (e) inappropriate chair heights, (f) high cabinets, (g) problems associated with stairs (e.g., lack of handrails, high steps, and worn and torn stair treads), (h) high gloss floors, and (i) high pile carpets (Archea, 1985; Brown, 1995; Connell and Wolf, 1997; Howe, 1994; Josephson et al., 1991; Lach et al., 1991; Perlin, 1992; Tinker, Askham, Glucksman, and Swift, 1991). Other factors that predispose the older adult to falls that are not categorized as intrinsic or extrinsic include: (a) the type and style of shoes worn, (b) behaviors or activities performed by the person, (c) a fear of falling, and (d) living alone (Archea, 1985; Craven and Bruno, 1986; Urton, 1991).

In research conducted by Lach et al. (1991), the current classification of falls (i.e., intrinsic and extrinsic factors) was reexamined to determine the reliability of this classification system. A random sample of 1,358 community-dwelling older adults living in the St. Louis area was monitored for falls. The results indicated that 366 falls had occurred during the year, and more importantly, 55 percent of these falls were due to extrinsic factors, while 31 percent were due to intrinsic factors. As this research suggests, falls are likely to occur due to environmental hazards. In fact, Reinsch et al. (1992b) and Northridge et al. (1995) both reiterated this fact and postulated that falls among healthy, community-dwelling older adults typically occur due to some built environmental factor. It is not until advanced age (i.e., over the age of 75) that intrinsic factors typically begin to play a stronger role in falling (Hindmarsh and Estes,1989). This fact is clearly reiterated in Table 1. Falls tend to occur indoors while the older adult is either in the bedroom or living room (Ashley et al., 1977; Cambell et al., 1990; Downtown and Andrews, 1991; Louis, 1983; Northridge et al., 1995; Reinsch, MacRae, Lachenbruch, and Tobis, 1992a; Reinsch et al., 1992b).

DESIGN ELEMENTS
THAT PREVENT FALLING

The risk of falling among older adults is greatly increased by environmental design hazards, and this risk is exacerbated in individuals with Parkinson's disease. Tremor, balance problems, stooped posture, shuffling gait, and muscle rigidity cause individuals with Parkinson's disease great hardship when manipulating their environment. Thus, the information that follows can be used as a check list in order to prevent some of the more common environmental hazards found within the home that often lead to falls (Hutton et al., 1997).

Floors

—Avoid bold patterns in carpets or other types of floor surfaces. Strong patterns can become disorienting to individuals with Parkinson's disease (Howe, 1994; Hutton et al., 1997; Perlin, 1992).
—Remove throw rugs, tack down carpet edges, and repair worn carpeting. Because of their shuffling gait, individuals with Parkinson's dis-

Table 1
Incidence and Causes/Risk Factors of Falling

Author	Sample	Incidence	Risk Factors
Ashley, Gryfe, and Amies (1977)	441 older adults living in a home for the aged (75 to 90 years)	668 per 1,000 persons per year	—female gender —occurred in bedroom or bathroom —majority occurred indoors
Louis (1983)	Institutionalized elderly (60 years and over)	4.05 falls per 1,000 patient days in facility A; 7.32 falls per 1,000 patient days in facility B	—male gender —increased age —majority occurred in resident bedroom
Gabell, Simons, and Nayak (1985)	100 community-dwelling subjects (65 years and over)	22 experienced falls during the year	—defective balance —footwear —disability —gait problems
Craven and Bruno (1986)	Convenience sample of community-dwelling older adults (65 years and older)	50% had fallen two to four times in past year	—advancing age —living alone —vision, balance, and neurological problems
Campbell, Borrie, Spears, et al. (1990)	761 subjects, over 70 community-dwelling	507 falls in last year	—majority occurred in bedroom —female gender —irregular foot path
Downtown and Andrews (1991)	203 people, 75 and older living in community (mean age 83)	42% in last year	—majority occurred in bedroom or living room —20% due to slip or trip —unstable knee joint —previous stroke —female gender —40% occurred outdoors —multifaceted causes
Lach et al. (1991)	Random sample of 1,358 community-dwelling older adults (mean age 74.8)	366 falls occurred during the year (30%)	—55% extrinsic —31% intrinsic (defective balance)
Reinsch, MacRae, Lachenbruch, and Tobis (1992b)	222 subjects recruited from senior centers (mean age 75.5)	29% had fallen in last year 50% had fallen in last two years	—environmental factors (bedroom and living room, getting out of bed, walking on uneven surface)

Table 1 (continued)
Incidence and Causes/Risk Factors of Falling

Tideiksaar (1992)	Community-dwelling older adults who had visited emergency room in last 17 months	49% had fallen previously	—environmental factors (unstable surfaces, slipping, and tripping)
Salgado, Lord, Packer, and Ehrlich (1994)	44 hospital patients who had fallen (mean age 80.7)	Not given	—cognitive impairment —incoordination —evidence of stroke —medications —balance problems
Northridge, Nevitt, Kelsey, and Link (1995)	Convenience sample of 325 older adults living in community	252 falls in last year	—46.8% of first falls were due to environmental factors —majority occurred in bedroom —storage problems —clutter —loose throw rugs
Connell and Wolf (1997)	15 older adults living in the community (70 to 81 years old)	Not given	—environmental factors (tripping over cords, stairs, high thresholds, avoiding hazards)
Woolley, Czaja, and Drury (1997)	Fallers versus nonfallers–22 older adults living in social services facility	Not given	—reduced step length —reduced stride length —increased stride time —decreased swing stance ratio —declines in balance —difficulty in descending stairs

ease can trip over the edges (Howe, 1994; Hutton et al., 1997; Northridge et al., 1995; Thompson, 1996; Ulfarsson and Robinson, 1994).

—Use non-skid wax on floors, avoid high-gloss floors, and use non-slip flooring (Howe, 1994; Perlin, 1992; Tideiksaar, 1986; Ulfarsson and Robinson, 1994; Thompson, 1996; Wilson, 1998).

—Remove high thresholds or transition strips that are often used between different floor materials (Howe, 1994; Hutton et al., 1997; Tideiksaar, 1986). If high thresholds are unavoidable, the edge should be clearly defined (e.g., use a contrasting tape along the edge of the threshold) (Hutton et al., 1997).

—Remove cords from the walking path, and remove small objects (e.g., books, sewing supplies, magazines, and newspapers) from the floor (Hutton et al., 1997; Ulfarsson and Robinson, 1994).

—Use carpet that is tightly woven and that has a low pile height (Hutton et al., 1997; Ulfarsson and Robinson, 1994).

Lighting

—Inadequate lighting and glare can cause individuals with Parkinson's disease to become confused, resulting in an increased propensity to fall (Anderson and Noell, 1994; Brown, 1995; Howe, 1994; Urton, 1991; Wilson, 1998). Glare may be prevented by (a) shielding light sources from the individual's view, (b) using indirect lighting, (c) avoiding exposed lamps, and (d) avoiding reflective materials (Behar, 1992; Williams, 1989).

—Provide adequate illumination for the task to be performed (Brent, Phillips, Brent, Gupta, and Degges, 1991; Howe, 1994; Thompson, 1996; Tideiksaar, 1986).

—Make certain that light switches are easily accessible (Howe, 1994). Provide high color contrast between the light switch and the wall.

—Use three-way light switches in both ends of a hallway. This will prevent a situation in which the older adult must walk an unlit corridor (Hutton et al., 1997).

Doors

—Use lever-type door handles that are much easier to grasp than door knobs (Howe, 1994).

—Provide at least 32 inches clear at the door opening so that assistive devices (i.e., walkers, canes, wheelchairs) have the necessary clearance (Howe, 1994).

—Doors to bathrooms should open out into the bedroom or hallway so when an individual does fall they do not block the door from opening (Howe, 1994).

Walls

—Provide enough color contrast between wall and floor surfaces for improved visibility.

Stairs

—Provide handrails on both sides of the stairwell. Handrails should extend 12 inches beyond the bottom step (Archea, 1985; Hutton et al., 1997; Howe, 1994; Urton, 1991).

—Provide adequate lighting in the stairwell and avoid glare. Use three-way switches at both ends of the stairwell (Archea, 1985) .

—Avoid high steps and worn stair treads (Hutton et al., 1997; Urton, 1991).

—High contrast should be provided to clearly define the stair edge (Hutton et al., 1997; Howe, 1994).

Bathrooms

—Use non-skid mats in the shower and the bathtub (Hutton et al., 1997).

—Equip shower stalls with grab bars, a bench, and a hand-held shower nozzle (Hutton et al., 1997).

—Provide grab bars to the side and behind the toilet (Hutton et al., 1997; Urton, 1991; Wilson, 1998).

—Avoid slippery floors (Urton, 1991).

—Provide a non-skid mat in front of the toilet to prevent slips when sitting or standing (Hutton et al., 1997).

Kitchens

—Avoid kitchen cabinets that are too high. This can result in a situation in which the older adult uses a step ladder or chair to reach items, causing a fall (Hutton et al., 1997; Urton, 1991).

Furniture

—Avoid tables with highly polished wood or glass surfaces that can become confusing and create glare in the interior environment (Howe, 1994).

—Avoid tables with a pedestal base. This is considered an unstable table type and will not support an individual's weight (Hutton et al., 1997).

—Furniture should have rounded edges to prevent injury (Howe, 1994).

—Provide high color contrast between furniture legs and floor surface. Individuals may trip over furniture legs when contrast is low.

—Use chairs with firm seat cushions and arms. Individuals with Parkinson's disease have difficulty getting out of chairs that are too low, have no arms, or that have extremely compliant seat cushions (Hutton et al., 1997; Howe, 1994).

—Furniture should be sturdy. Many individuals with Parkinson's disease use furniture to help them get up from a seated position or to steady themselves while walking through the house.

—Consider removing your coffee table. Coffee tables not only lead to falls, but they can also cause severe injury when a fall does occur (Hutton et al., 1997).

—When selecting a chair, make sure your feet rest firmly on the floor when you are seated. This allows for good balance when rising and sitting (Hutton et al., 1997).

Bedrooms

—Consider installing handrails on both sides of the bed. This will not only prevent a fall while sleeping, but will also aid the individual with Parkinson's disease in getting out of the bed (Hutton et al., 1997).

SUMMARY

The population of older adults in the United States will continue to increase as advances in medical science and technology allow individuals to live longer. Unfortunately, these advances come with a price. Although individuals can expect to live longer, longer life expectancies cannot always be associated with good health. Many older adults will suffer from age-related changes such as visual impairments, hearing impairments, degeneration of tactile sensitivity, loss of muscle strength, and Parkinson's disease. All of these age-related changes put the older adult at risk for balance and gait problems that can result in a fall.

Falling is a common problem among older adults; 30 percent of community-dwelling older adults fall annually (Brown, 1995; Tideiksaar,

1989; Tinetti and Williams, 1998). Even though many of these falls are due to intrinsic factors that are associated with aging or disease, falls due to environmental design factors are more common among the "young old" (i.e., those individuals under the age of 75). Moreover, the majority of falls tend to occur inside the older adult's home. Despite the fact that the built environment is mentioned as a factor contributing to falls, many older adults continue to live in homes with numerous hazardous conditions. This is unfortunate when, as illustrated in this chapter, interior design modifications can easily be made in order to improve safety within the home. As individuals grow older, the need for changes in the home environment should be dictated by the physical and mental capabilities of the person. Safety should be a first priority.

REFERENCES

American Association of Retired Persons. (1994). *A Profile of Older Americans* (Issue Brief No. PF3049 1294). Washington, D.C.: Author.

Anderson, L., and Noell, E. (1994). "The aging population: Everyone would benefit from a fresh approach." *Lighting Design and Application* 24(3):32–36.

Ashley, M. J., Gryfe, C. I., and Amies, A. (1977). "A longitudinal study of falls in an elderly population: Some circumstances of falling." *Age and Ageing* 6:211–20.

Archea, J. C. (1985). "Environmental factors associated with stair accidents by the elderly." *Clinics in Geriatric Medicine* 1:555–69.

Behar, S. (1992). "Making accessibility easy on the eye." *The Construction Specifier* 45(6):114–19.

Brawley, E. C. (1997). *Designing for Alzheimer's Disease: Strategies for Creating Better Care Environments.* New York: John Wiley & Sons.

Brent, R. S., Phillips, R. G., Brent, E. E., Gupta, M. K., and Degges, S. R. (1991). "Older adults residing in their own home: Prioritizing housing inadequacies." *Housing and Society* 18(1):25–33.

Brown, D. I. (1995). "Falls in elderly population: A look at incidence, risks, healthcare costs, and preventative strategies." *Rehabilitation Nursing* 20(2):84–89.

Cambell, A. J., Borrie, M. J., Spears, G. F., Jackson, S. L., Brown, J. S., and Fitzgerald, J. L. (1990). "Circumstances and consequences of falls experienced by a community population 70 years and over during a prospective study." *Age and Ageing* 19:136–41.

Connell, B. R., and Wolf, S. L. (1997). "Environmental and behavioral circumstances associated with falls at home among healthy elderly individuals." *Archives of Physical Medicine Rehabilitation* 78(2): 179–86.

Craven, R., and Bruno, P. (1986). "Teach the elderly to prevent falls." *Journal of Gerontological Nursing* 12(8):27–33.

Creasey, R., and Broe, G. A. (1993). "Prescribing for the elderly: Parkinson's disease." *The Medical Journal of Australia* 159:249–53.

Downtown, J. H., and Andrews, K. (1991). "Prevalence, characteristics and factors associated with falls among the elderly living at home." *Aging* 3:219–28.

Duvoisin, R. C., and Sage, J. (1996). *Parkinson's Disease: A Guide for Patient and Family.* Philadelphia: Lippincott-Raven Publishers.

Gabell, A., Simons, M. A., and Nayak, U. S. L. (1985). "Falls in the healthy elderly: Predisposing causes." *Ergonomics* 28:965–75.

Hindmarsh, J. J., and Estes, E. H. (1989). "Falls in older persons." *Archives of Internal Medicine* 149:2217–22.

Howe, J. S. (1994). "Preventing falls through environmental assessment." *Nursing Homes* 43:10–19.

Hutton, J. T., Elias, J. W., Shroyer, J. L., and Curry, Z. (1997). *Preventing Falls: A Defensive Approach.* Lubbock, Tx.: Neurology Research and Education Center.

Josephson, K. R., Fabacher, D. A., and Rubenstein, D. A. (1991). "Home safety and fall prevention." *Clinics in Geriatric Medicine* 7:707–31.

Klawans, H. L., and Topel, J. L. (1974). "Parkinsonism as a falling sickness." *Journal of the American Medical Association* 230:1555–57.

Lach, H. W., Reed, A. T., Arfken, C. L., Miller, J. P., Paige, G. D., Birge, S. J., and Peck, W. A. (1991). "Falls in the elderly: Reliability of a classification system." *Journal of American Geriatrics Society* 39:197–202.

Louis, M. (1983). "Falls and their causes." *Journal of Gerontological Nursing* 9(3):142–56.

Nevitt, M. C., Cummings, S. R., and Hudes, E. S. (1991). "Risk factors for injurious falls: A prospective study." *Journal of Gerontology: Medical Sciences* 46:M164–M170.

Northridge, M. E., Nevitt, N. C., Kelsey, J. L., and Link, B. (1995). "Home hazards and falls in the elderly: The role of health and functional status." *American Journal of Public Health* 85:509–15.

Pearce, J. M. (1992). *Parkinson's Disease and Its Management.* New York: Oxford University Press.

Perlin, E. (1992). "Preventing falls in the elderly." *Postgraduate Medicine* 91(8):237–44.

Pirkl, J. J. (1994). *Transgenerational Design: Products for an Aging Population*. New York: Van Nostrand Reinhold.

Reinsch, S., MacRae, P., Lachenbruch, P. A., and Tobis, J. S. (1992a). "Attempts to prevent falls and injury: A prospective community study." *The Gerontologist* 12:450–56.

Reinsch, S., MacRae, P., Lachenbruch, P. A., and Tobis, J. S. (1992b). "Why do healthy older adults fall? Behavioral and environmental risks." *Physical & Occupational Therapy in Geriatrics* 11(1):1–15.

Salgado, R., Lord, S. R., Packer, J., and Ehrlich, F. (1994). "Factors associated with falling in elderly hospital patients." *Gerontology* 40:325–31.

Shroyer, J. L. (1994). "Recommendations for environmental design research correlating falls and the physical environment." *Experimental Aging Research* 20:303–309.

Thompson, P. G. (1996). "Preventing falls in the elderly at home: A community-based program." *Medical Journal of Australia* 164:530–32.

Tideiksaar, R. (1986). "Preventing falls: Home hazard checklists to help older patients protest themselves." *Geriatrics* 41(5):26–28.

Tideiksaar, R. (1989). *Falling in Older Age: Its Prevention and Treatment*. New York: Springer.

Tideiksaar, R. (1992). "Falls among the elderly: A community prevention program." *American Journal of Public Health* 82:892–93.

Tinetti, M. E. (1989). "Instability and falling elderly patients." *Seminars in Neurology* 9(1):39–45.

Tinetti, M. E., and Williams, C. S. (1998). "The effects of falls and fall injuries on functioning community-dwelling older persons." *Journal of Gerontology: Medical Sciences* 53A:M112–M119.

Tinker, A., Askham, J., Glucksman, E., and Swift, C. (1991). "Falls to elderly people: Housing and other environmental risk factors." *Housing Review* 40(3):70–72.

Ulfarsson, J., and Robinson, B. E. (1994). "Preventing falls and fractures." *Journal of the Florida Medical Association* 81:763–67.

Urton, M. M. (1991). "A community home inspection approach to preventing falls among the elderly." *Public Health Reports* 106(2):192–195.

Williams, M. A. (1989). "Physical environment of the intensive care unit and elderly patients." *Critical Care Nursing Quarterly* 12(1):52–60.

Wilson, E. B. (1998). "Preventing patient falls." *AACN Clinical Issues* 9(1):100–108.

Woolley, S. M., Czaja, S. J., and Drury, C. G. (1997). "An assessment of falls in elderly men and women." *Journal of Gerontology: Medical Sciences* 52A:M80–M87.

12

Surgical Treatments for Parkinson's Disease

Bhupesh H. Dihenia

INTRODUCTION

Parkinson's disease is a neurodegenerative disorder characterized by loss of dopamine-producing cells in the substantia nigra. Due to the lack of dopamine, there is some malfunctioning of the deep brain circuitry called the basal ganglia. This malfunction manifests clinically as slowness of movements (bradykinesia), resting tremor, rigidity, and postural instability. Fortunately, there are many pharmacological interventions which, in early stages of the disease, help significantly. Unfortunately, the disease continues to progress, and the antiparkinsonian medication treatment may be complicated by debilitating side effects such as dyskinesias, neuropsychiatric difficulties, and motor fluctuations. Although there are many new medications currently available to help with these symptoms, the disease may progress to the point where pharmacological intervention alone is sometimes not satisfactory.

There are two proven surgical interventions for medically intractable Parkinson's disease: pallidotomy and deep brain stimulation. Currently, there are also two ongoing research surgical interventions known as nerve cell transplantation and nerve growth factors.

Surgical intervention for medically intractable Parkinson's disease was initially attempted in the early years of the 1900s. Unfortunately, there was not a very good understanding of neural anatomy at that time, and various targets were sought based on minimal scientific merit. In the 1950s, Dr. Lars Leksell performed pallidotomy on 81 patients and studied them scientifically. Approximately 80 percent of his patients experienced complete tremor alleviation. Unfortunately, a significant number of them also developed some visual field deficits and hemiparesis (paralysis on one side). With the advent of levodopa, the main ingredient in Sinemet, the interest in surgical intervention diminished.

Some interest in doing surgery to improve tremor remained among physicians treating Parkinson's disease. In the late 1960s, thalamotomy (lesioning another nuclei in the deep brain) was studied. This improved the tremor significantly, but made no improvement on the slowness of movements. Thalamotomy also caused a worsening of speech.

Dr. Lauri Laiten continued to systematically study pallidotomies. He was able to report significant improvement in the parkinsonian motor signs as well as benefit the drug-induced dyskinesias. Currently, the pallidotomy is an approved treatment for medically intractable Parkinson's disease.

PALLIDOTOMY

Pallidotomy is performed two ways. In stereotactic pallidotomy, a head frame is placed on the patient and secured to the skull. An MRI (magnetic resonance imaging) scan is performed, and a lesion site in the globus pallidus is selected based on anatomy only. An electrode is then placed in the brain in that area which has been selected by the MRI guidance to be ablated. This procedure works relatively well.

Another way of performing pallidotomy is using microelectrode guidance. Once again the head frame is placed on the patient, an MRI is taken, and a microelectrode is inserted into the brain. The microelectrode then records single cells and helps make a map of the patient's brain. The individual regions of the brain have different firing patterns which translate into different sound patterns. A particular region called globus pallidus interni, which is the final outflow for the deep brain circuit basal ganglia, is then located by monitoring and testing different sites within the brain. When the correct site is located, the tip of the microelectrode is heated and this region is then lesioned. There is significant improvement of motor function on the side of the body opposite that from which the brain pallidotomy is performed. There is immediate amelioration of the tremor and reduction of rigidity, as well as improved slowness of movements.

The key to performing a pallidotomy is to ensure that the optic tract is not damaged. The optic tract carries the visual information from the eyes to the back of the head, where the information is actually interpreted. The optic tract runs near the globus pallidus interni. The internal capsule, which carries the nerve fibers from the cortex of the brain, where movements are initiated, to the spinal cord and into the muscles for executing the movements, is also located near the globus pallidus interni. These two regions (optic tract and internal capsule) need to be defined during the pallidotomy so that lesions are not made too near to them. The consequences of interrupting these tracts include visual field deficits as well as hemiparesis.

There are many centers around the country that are currently performing the pallidotomy successfully. It provides an excellent alternative for patients with drug-induced dyskinesia or dystonia, as well as for patients with intractable motor fluctuations or tremor. Unfortunately, postural instability is a symptom that is little helped by the pallidotomy.

DEEP BRAIN STIMULATION

Chronic deep brain stimulation (DBS) has been used for treatment of parkinsonian tremor as well as familial essential tremor. The deep brain stimulator is essentially a pacemaker of the brain. It has been approved by the FDA to be inserted into a particular lesion of the thalamus. It will significantly improve tremor, including a nonparkinsonian tremor called familial or essential tremor. Unfortunately, deep brain stimulation does not improve the other cardinal symptoms of Parkinson's disease. The deep brain stimulator is inserted into a particular nucleus of the thalamus and then the power source is implanted above the clavicle. This pulse generator (pacemaker) is connected to the electrode by a wire which runs under the skin. The pacemaker can then be programmed by a computer to determine frequency and amplitude of the output. The output then apparently confuses the thalamus's own firing pattern and the tremor is significantly improved.

The advantages of deep brain stimulation over the thalamotomy are several. There is no destruction of brain tissue with deep brain stimulation, and therefore it is completely reversible. Hopefully in the future, when better treatments and possible cures are available, the deep brain stimulator can be removed and better options can be pursued.

Currently, the deep brain stimulator is only approved to be placed in the thalamus, but there are clinical research trials ongoing for placing a deep brain stimulator in other regions of the brain, such as the globus pallidus and subthalamic nucleus. Basically, the researchers are attempting to determine whether deep brain stimulation can be used to interfere with the basal ganglia circuit at some point at which it can help the parkinsonian symptoms.

NERVE GROWTH FACTORS

Research using nerve growth factors—pharmacological agents that enhance the survival and growth of nerve cells—has begun in Parkinson's disease patients within the last year. No data yet exist for results in humans. One such nerve growth factor, GDNF (glial-derived neurotrophic factor), is currently being tested in humans for safety, tolerability, and potential benefit for Parkinson's disease. Nerve growth factors have shown significant improvement in the MPTP animal model of Parkinson's disease, and have also significantly improved the symptoms of Parkinson's disease in monkeys and rats. This improvement has led to significant enthusiasm for extending the research to humans. Extensive research testing is currently underway.

In the surgical procedure for nerve growth factor, a neurosurgeon attaches a frame to the patient's head to aid in identifying the specific brain area into which to place a catheter. The catheter is placed through the brain tissue into the fluid-filled space called the lateral ventricle. The catheter is connected to the delivery port inserted just underneath the skin on the skull. Two weeks after surgery, the study material, GDNF, is then injected into the delivery port, from which it reaches the lateral ventricle. It is hoped that nerve growth factor will allow the survival and even the generation of dopamine-producing cells. A more recent experimental approach is to infuse the GDNF via a continuous pump that is imbedded in the abdomen or chest. The pump infuses the GDNF via a catheter to the ventricle of the brain.

NERVE CELL TRANSPLANTATION

Nerve cell transplantation—implantating brain cells that produce dopamine—is also an experimental procedure. Various types of dopamine-producing cells have been tested, such as adrenal cells, human fetal cells, and pig fetal cells. The results of these studies are yet to be seen, and it remains more controversial than other procedures. Currently, increased numbers of fetal neurons are surviving the grafting, reinnervating parts of the brain, and mediating some clinically relevant benefits. Extensive research is ongoing in this field.

The patients who are qualified for the surgical interventions are those in whom the medications are no longer controlling the symptoms adequately. To qualify, the Parkinson's disease patient should not have any dementia; otherwise, surgery is contraindicated. Pallidotomy as well as deep brain stimulation predominantly help the side of the body opposite from the brain surgery. Pallidotomy has been shown to result in a profound improvement of drug-induced dyskinesias and dystonias. But though the surgeries improve some symptoms significantly, they do not alter the natural progression of the disease, and symptoms will again get worse with time.

SUMMARY

In summary, there are numerous pharmacological interventions to help the clinical symptoms of Parkinson's disease, and many more medications are currently undergoing research trials. Unfortunately, due to the natural progression of the disease, patients develop symptoms which are not ameliorated by medication alone, and the medications themselves may cause side effects. With better understanding of the pathophysiology and the circuitry of the deep brain, surgical interventions have added to the treatment of Parkinson's disease. With technological advancements such as mapping deep brain regions by monitoring individual cells, researchers have advanced surgical treatment significantly. Currently, pallidotomy and deep brain stimulation of the thalamus are approved surgical interventions. Clinical research trials are ongoing for deep brain stimulation of the globus pallidus and subthalamic nucleus. Trials for nerve growth factors as well as nerve cell transplantations are also ongoing. These developments encourage optimism for the future treatment of Parkinson's disease.

13

Cognitive Changes Associated with Parkinson's Disease

Charles R. Walker

INTRODUCTION

When James Parkinson first described "the shaking palsy" in 1817, he noted that the illness was characterized by a number of distinct physical symptoms with "the senses and intellect being uninjured." Indeed, Parkinson's disease is much more widely known for its motor symptoms than for producing changes in mental abilities. Nevertheless, a variety of alterations in thinking and memory have been associated with Parkinson's disease for many patients, to the extent that there is now a sizeable volume of research on the subject.

The purpose of this chapter is twofold. The first goal is to acquaint the reader with what has become known about cognitive changes in Parkinson's disease through research and clinical observation, including the relationship between Parkinson's disease and dementia (severe memory disorder and cognitive dysfunction). Secondly, suggestions for dealing with these problems and the role of neurorehabilitation are also discussed.

Cognition is the broad term generally used to refer to the processes by which the brain (1) manipulates information, both newly derived from the senses as well as recalled from previous experience, and (2) plans and executes intentional behavior. Cognition therefore includes those unseen mental efforts we commonly refer to as "thinking," as well as other operations such as perception, attentional control, memory functions, and certain aspects of motor planning and control that normally seem essentially effortless and automatic.

Attempts to study the cognitive changes associated with Parkinson's disease have met with multiple challenges. First, Parkinson's disease most frequently occurs in persons who are in their sixties or beyond, and who are thus subject to the cognitive effects of the aging process. Unhappily, many of us are learning from personal experience that aging alone can and does produce some alterations in our mental abilities. Research must be designed so as not to confuse normal changes associated with aging with the effects of disease. Also, it is important to control for the effects of other conditions that become more prevalent with increasing age and that might be present—though as yet undetected—in some research subjects, such as cardiovascular disease or early Alzheimer's disease. Furthermore, Parkinson's disease is not a static condition; it typically is progressive, and patients with the illness vary greatly in terms of disability. Thus, some studies that take a one-time measurement of a sample of patients may fail to allow us to appreciate differences occurring during the course of the illness. The motor difficulties associated with Parkinson's disease confound the results of standard tests for perceptual motor abilities, as motor problems to some degree can mask the visuospatial processing and planning abilities of a patient. Additionally, Parkinson's disease is associated with anxiety and depression, emotional conditions known to exert a negative influence on performance on standardized tests. Finally, some of the medications used by patients with Parkinson's disease may affect various aspects of test performance as well. While these factors have complicated the systematic study of the cognitive effects of Parkinson's disease, much has nevertheless been learned.

It is important for the reader to understand that persons with Parkinson's disease are as varied as any other group of people, and neuropsychological studies have failed to identify any consistent ability profile that reliably describes the effects of this illness for any one individual patient. This is hardly surprising, as other research has determined that many causative factors can lead to the constellation of problems identified with this illness. Nevertheless, some cognitive features are commonly observed. Do not forget, however, that at an individual level the effects of Parkinson's disease on cognitive ability can range from rather minimal, generalized effects on thinking and recall efficiency— effects that may be insignificantly different from aging effects alone—to significant impairment appropriately classified as dementia. In fact, for the purposes of discussion as well as research, it is useful to separate the topic of dementia from discussion of the other cognitive effects of Parkinson's disease, as those patients who develop dementia appear to constitute a distinct and separate subgroup of patients.

Various studies have estimated that upward of 50 percent of Parkinson's disease patients suffer from measurable changes in cognition, with such changes seen more commonly in patients who are older and/or whose duration of disease is longer. Not surprisingly, there is also a relationship between severity of Parkinson's disease and the degree of cognitive dysfunction observed. None of these relationships are exceedingly strong, however, and exceptions are often seen. For example, some patients in their eighties with longstanding and relatively severe Parkinson's disease symptoms show no effects on their thinking and memory abilities beyond what one would expect from aging effects alone.

GENERALIZED VERSUS SPECIFIC EFFECTS

Neuropsychologists and neurologists often characterize the influences of various conditions affecting the brain as producing *generalized effects* versus *specific effects*. Generalized effects, as the name implies, tend to impact virtually all aspects of a person's cognitive functioning. Aging, for example, appears to produce mostly generalized effects on information-processing abilities, impacting to some extent one's speed of performance, recall for multiple types of information, thinking speed, and so forth. In contrast, specific effects are changes noted in more isolated aspects of behavior, suggesting dysfunction in specific information-processing systems. These systems are often fairly well understood in terms of anatomical regions or connections between regions, and their disruption can be reliably associated with the failure of certain parts of the brain to function normally. Some diseases or injuries—for example, certain small, localized strokes—often lead to problems affecting certain abilities such as speech or motor control of one side of the body, with little impact on other abilities. Parkinson's disease appears to result in both types of effects, though in general many of the difficulties seen appear related to dysfunction in the anterior, or frontal, portion of the brain.

CRYSTALLIZED VERSUS FLUID INTELLECTUAL ABILITIES

Another useful concept is the notion of *crystallized* versus *fluid* intellectual abilities. Some cognitive abilities are heavily practiced due to almost constant use, such as basic language functions, social graces, and the retention and easy recall of a fundamental knowledge base. These abilities have been described as "crystallized" or "overlearned." While catastrophic illnesses or physical injuries to the brain can disrupt these types of abilities, slowly progressive illnesses tend to spare these functions over time. Parkinson's disease patients generally do not show significant decline with respect to their crystallized mental abilities. In contrast, however, impairments can be seen in such patients with respect to their so-called "fluid" abilities: the ability to rapidly adapt to new situations and circumstances, and to apply knowledge and problem-solving to novel situations and challenges requiring high-level mental conceptualization and immediate adaptive actions or plans. Parkinson's disease patients thus may continue to function well at work or at home in activities quite familiar to them and in which they have been engaged for many years, but they may experience a surprising level of difficulty when faced with unfamiliar challenges or tasks, or are required to adapt to a new environment or routine.

CORTICAL VERSUS SUBCORTICAL FEATURES

Most people are familiar with the term "gray matter," a description of the cortical tissue of the brain where thinking and information processing occurs. "Gray matter" is a description of the outermost layer of the brain—the part that would be visible if an intact brain were viewed from the outside. This wrinkled surface of the brain is called the *cerebral cortex*. Actually, this layer of tissue consists of the cell bodies of the *neurons*, or nerve cells, that make up the *cerebrum*, or higher brain centers. The bulk of the underlying brain has been called "white matter," a term aptly describing the appearance of tissues composed of projections from the cell bodies called *axons,* which are covered in a whitish substance known as *myelin.* Myelin serves to insulate the axons in much the same way as the insulation coating on wires we use in electrical circuits. Since nerve cells communicate with one another via electrochemical means, it is not surprising that the brain in many ways resembles an incredibly complex computer with interconnections between many different circuits.

Buried within the cerebrum are other gray matter structures known as the *basal ganglia.* These structures are important in the control of movement. The motor difficulties associated with Parkinson's disease arise from damage to neurons in the basal ganglia. Because these problems occur in portions of the brain below the cortex, Parkinson's disease is often referred to as a *subcortical* brain disease, though some aspects of the functioning of the cortex are likely affected as well.

If cognition occurs in the cortex, then why can a subcortical disease affect cognition? This has been the subject of considerable debate in the past, but it is known that the functioning of the cortex can be affected by damage to important underlying structures. Dysfunction of two other deep gray-matter structures, the *locus coeruleus* and the *nucleus basalis of Meynert*, has been implicated in affecting cognitive abilities, as these structures appear to serve as important "relay centers" or "connecting hubs" for important parts of the rich network of connections in the brain. Nevertheless, the cognitive and behavioral effects of subcortical disease or injury are somewhat different from what is typically seen in *cortical* diseases, such as Alzheimer's disease. For the interested reader, there are sources of more detailed information regarding these fascinating brain systems listed at the end of this chapter.

GENERAL THINKING ABILITIES AND MENTAL CONTROL

What, then, are the observable changes most often seen in Parkinson's disease patients with cognitive impairments? One commonly observed cognitive change associated with Parkinson's disease is called *bradyphrenia*, which refers to the slowing of thinking processes. It has been noted that *some* Parkinson's disease patients develop slowness in their ability to think and respond that mimics, interestingly, the quality of their motor problems. Besides experiencing a slowing down of thinking per se, patients often demonstrate problems in initiating their thought processes or their verbal responses. Furthermore, they may tend to become rather "fixed" mentally on a particular idea or concern and have difficulty shifting their perspective or point of view. They may also *perseverate*, or persist, with an idea or mental "set" from one situation to another where the idea is incorrect or inappropriate. This can lead to frustration for both the patient and caregiver. *Cognitive inflexibility* is the term often used to describe this set of cognitive difficulties, all of which likely result from changes in frontal lobe functioning in the brain. It is easy to see how these types of cognitive difficulties can interact with and exacerbate certain emotional qualities, such as anxiety and depression. It requires a certain amount of cognitive flexibility to generate alternatives and solutions in order to become "unstuck" from troublesome situations or other daily problems.

Those Parkinson's disease patients with cognitive features may also have problems in complex attentional control. While their basic attentional processes are intact, they appear to have problems with complex attentional demands—that is, in situations requiring the ability to simultaneously pay attention to several things at once. This may relate to problems in organizing an internal strategy for maintaining their attention, or it may be the result of difficulties in continually shifting attention. They sometimes show difficulties with planning and sequencing some motor activities, a problem called *dyspraxia*. There appears to be a more general problem with conceptualizing events in a time sequence, as such patients generally have problems on tests requiring them to organize simple story pictures in a correct sequence, though other judgment factors are also required on such tests.

The ability to conceptualize information at an abstract level has long been associated with frontal lobe functioning, but also has been noted to become impaired in many instances of brain injury where the frontal lobe does not appear to have been specifically involved. Neuropsychologists therefore consider deficits in this particular ability to involve an inability of the frontal lobe to perform optimally, but the reason in any individual case may not be due to frontal lobe dysfunction per se, but rather may relate to problems with information being input to the frontal lobe from other areas of the brain. Parkinson's disease patients with cognitive deficits usually show considerable difficulty in thinking abstractly and in forming mental concepts for complex ideas. It seems possible that these difficulties may be a result from faulty input to the frontal lobe, as well as changes in the frontal lobe itself. More research is needed to elucidate the different factors that contribute to this type of deficit.

VISUOSPATIAL ABILITIES

Much of our intellectual abilities in thinking and problem-solving involve the use of verbal ability, either for expression of ideas or formulation of solutions. But other skills that involve processing and analyzing visual information and thinking about qualities such as size, position, and space are largely independent of our language abilities. The ability to make judgments about how a disassembled item might be put together, making size or other comparisons between objects, or even more basic visual processing such as recognizing faces are all examples of visuospatial abilities.

Patients with Parkinson's disease appear more vulnerable to changes with respect to visuospatial abilities than with verbal abilities. Problems are sometimes seen in basic visuospatial tasks such as those requiring assembly of objects or recreation of visual patterns from constituent parts (for example, arranging colored blocks in order to duplicate a model), but problems are also seen in the ability to remember visual information.

MEMORY

Some memory impairment is also frequently seen in Parkinson's disease patients without dementia. However, in these cases, the memory disturbance is not severe enough, nor is it accompanied by other cognitive deficits of sufficient degree, to be considered dementia. Research on memory has demonstrated that our memory abilities involve many different and often relatively independent processing functions. For this reason, memory can be affected for certain types of information and not for others. Again, memory is one of those abilities known to change with aging, but the extent of change varies from one person to another and can also be subject to situational variables such as emotional state. The stress of being evaluated can even interfere with memory performance!

Most conditions leading to memory impairment demonstrate changes that are counterintuitive to most people. It seems logical that information learned long ago would be the most vulnerable to disruption and loss due to pathological changes in the brain, while experiences or facts that have been recently learned would be "fresher" and thus easier to recall. In fact, the opposite is true. Old information is stored in the brain in a manner that is much more resistant to loss from injury or disease, while new information is much more vulnerable to loss. In fact, this is one of the lines of evidence that has led researchers and memory theorists to conclude that the brain "moves" or reprocesses remembered information through several stages over the course of time, and these processes lead to greater and greater consolidation of those memories. Even patients with dementia often have little trouble recalling their past, such as their adolescence or early adulthood, but may have grave difficulty remembering a recent meal or whether they have taken their medication. All of us, in our daily lives, experience short-term memory failures from time to time.

In addition to the length of time since one was exposed to information that has been remembered, there are other important distinctions to be made in the types of information we remember. In particular, there are two major types of memory, *declarative memory* and *procedural memory*. Declarative memory refers to memory for facts and events, and can be further subdivided into *episodic memory*, or memory for events that have been experienced, and *factual memory*, or memory for learned facts. Retrieval processes for these types of memory are organized differently as well. For example, factual memories are organized in such a way that people generally know almost immediately whether they do or do not know something, and often whether they knew or did not know the information in the past, regardless of whether they can retrieve it presently.

We also make a distinction between memory problems due to a failure to successfully store the information somewhere in the brain, and difficulties due to problems in retrieval of stored information. Some studies of memory function in Parkinson's disease patients have appeared to indicate that memory problems in this illness stem principally from impairment of the control and retrieval strategies used to "call up" information from memory, rather than problems with encoding information, but most studies implicate the secondary and consolidation processes as defective. Regardless, learning of more rapidly paced, complex information can show impairment due to problems in mentally organizing and associating the information for effective recall. It appears that the rate of new information presentation can exceed a patient's rate of processing and thus produce an apparent memory deficit actually related to processing speed.

Most patients with mild memory problems are able to use cues to enhance or stimulate their recall of recently acquired information, suggesting that memory devices may be quite helpful with this population. Immediate auditory memory is usually intact for age, and the ability to recognize information as familiar or previously learned versus new is not greatly different than what is seen in normal aging control subjects.

Interestingly, some researchers have proposed a "cognitive subtype" of Parkinson's disease that demonstrates memory impairment only, without other thinking difficulties. More research is needed to clarify whether there may indeed be subtypes of Parkinson's disease differentiated by different patterns of cognitive and memory strengths and weaknesses.

CHANGES IN LANGUAGE-RELATED ABILITIES AND PARKINSON'S DISEASE

It is difficult to separate language issues from general cognitive issues, but certain difficulties seen in Parkinson's disease impact expressive communication. A common clinical finding among these patients is a change in vocal quality called *hypophonia*, which is characterized by a weak, soft voice that can be difficult to hear. Similarly, many Parkinson's disease patients will demonstrate handwriting described as *micrographia* (literally, "small writing"). Broader expressive difficulties sometimes observed are classified generally as *hypokinetic dysarthria*. These changes include a tendency to speak in a monotone fashion, with little variation in loudness or pitch of the voice, reduced use of vocal stress for emphasis, and use of short phrases. Consonant sounds may be imprecisely articulated, and sometimes speech is produced in "segmented rushes," or short bursts of words with inappropriate (agrammatical) pausing between these bursts.

Parkinson's disease patients have been found to have increased difficulty with retrieving names for both other people and for common objects. They also have problems on some tasks that require them to generate language under time pressure—for example, to name as many foods as possible, or as many words that begin with a specific letter. Such tasks relate to the construct called *verbal fluency*, a language feature usually associated with anterior structures on the left side of the brain.

Other common features of Parkinson's disease impact communication ability. For example, many patients exhibit a mask-like, unexpressive facial expression (*mask-like facies*), and they often reduce their use of gestures and other body language features. These changes in nonverbal aspects of language can compromise communication ability.

DEMENTIA AND PARKINSON'S DISEASE

Perhaps one of the more common fears of older Americans is the worry that their memory and thinking abilities will dramatically fail, and most persons have known people directly or indirectly who experienced dramatic loss of memory or other abilities in their later years. It has been estimated that more than 90 different disorders can result in a dementia syndrome. Parkinson's disease patients are not immune to developing other conditions as well, and memory loss in a Parkinson's disease patient requires the same careful clinical work-up to exclude other treatable causes that would be afforded any other patient. While Parkinson's disease patients do face an increased risk that they may develop a dementia syndrome, it is far from a certainty that such difficulties will arise. A recent study estimates that less than 30 percent of Parkinson's disease patients are found to experience either cognitive or memory difficulties of sufficient severity to cause pronounced difficulties in their lives.

Estimates of the rate of occurrence of dementia in Parkinson's disease have varied greatly from study to study, and making such estimates is difficult because the prevalence of dementia increases in general as age increases. Dementia itself can vary in how it is defined from one study to another, and by most definitions it can range from mild to severe. Studies report estimates ranging from 15 to 50 percent of Parkinson's disease patients who develop dementia, with a value of approximately 20 percent appearing to be a fairly reliable estimate derived from some of the best designed studies. This also resonates with findings related to other issues such as debility. Importantly, it is not clear that dementia in Parkinson's disease is always progressive in the same manner as more widely known and observed dementing illnesses, particularly Alzheimer's disease—a condition whose name is erroneously used by many people as a synonym for "dementia." Dementia in Parkinson's disease is *not necessarily* characterized by the same features or the same clinical course as Alzheimer's disease, though a relationship between these illnesses appears to exist. It does appear that the number of Parkinson's disease patients who are found to have post-mortem evidence of the physical manifestations of Alzheimer's disease represents a higher percentage of those patients than is found in the general population.

IMPLICATIONS FOR CAREGIVERS

As mentioned earlier in this chapter, it is important to realize that every patient is an individual with his or her own unique personality, strengths, and weaknesses in terms of abilities. Changes in abilities occur to everyone as we get older, and not every alteration noted in an older person represents the effects of disease or is a harbinger of progressive, serious decline. Though a sizeable proportion of Parkinson's disease patients will face changes in their cognitive and memory abilities, they can benefit from reassurance that, in many cases, these changes may be limited in degree and will not necessarily be markedly progressive. A sense of humor and a realistic outlook provide real help in coping with changing functions, whether due to age alone or the additional impact of a disease such as Parkinson's.

Because of the differences seen in abilities involving crystallized versus fluid skills, it is important to realize that even those patients with rather clear-cut cognitive problems are likely to be able to function independently in many situations. This is particularly true in circumstances involving familiar challenges and application of years of previous experience with the same general type of task or problem. Patients, particularly younger ones, may be able to continue working productively when their physical functioning allows and their skills are equal to the task. Nevertheless, it is often not the patient but rather family members or co-workers who first realize when the patient is having problems. Difficulties involving cognitive flexibility can cause patients to have difficulties appreciating differences between similar situations that call for different approaches—for example, in business dealings and decisions. They may show signs of a fixed mental set by trying one favorite or most common approach to an array of different problems, sometime quite inappropriately. When necessary, formal neuropsychological testing of abilities may help answer specific questions about a patient's current functioning and the appropriateness of continuing with specific responsibilities versus relinquishing control in some aspects of their lives. The neuropsychologist can sometimes assist both the patient and family in adapting to changes in roles and responsibilities.

Patience on the part of caregivers is important, as many patients indeed continue to have intact thinking abilities but may require additional time to formulate their verbal responses or actions. Giving the slowed patient time to respond in conversation is important to prevent frustration, anxiety, and dependency. Patients with frontal lobe difficulties are often able to benefit from having someone else segment a complex problem into a series of basic steps which he or she can then tackle one step at a time, often with success. They also may need help to organize their environment, particularly if they have not been especially organized in the past. This applies not only to organizing items in the home, but organizing time into a somewhat predictable routine when possible.

Memory aids can be helpful when needed. Making lists, writing in a notebook, using a wall calendar, and/or dictating into a pocket recorder can become helpful habits that increase the patient's self-reliance and decrease the need to depend on others. Gentle cueing or prompting to use such aids, rather than automatically "doing the work" for the patient, facilitates adoption of these systems.

Driving is important to almost all adults, but memory, visuospatial processing ability, and processing speed are all required to drive safely. Again, concerns frequently occur to persons other than the patient, and unfortunately the threat of losing the privilege to drive can be so great as to cause great interpersonal difficulties between an impaired patient and his family or caregivers. Nonetheless, it is an important responsibility to safeguard not only the patient from her or his own actions, but to protect other innocents as well. Again, driving evaluations can be completed at many outpatient rehabilitation centers or by occupational therapy services. Since driver's license renewal requirements vary greatly from state to state, one cannot necessarily rely on the state motor vehicle department to always appropriately withhold a license from a citizen, nor do all persons without licenses cease to drive!

Perhaps as many as 50 percent of Parkinson's disease patients suffer depression and anxiety associated with their illness. These emotional conditions, particularly depression, can sometimes produce cognitive symptoms that mimic early dementia. It is important to realize that these problems can be reversed with appropriate treatment of the emotional disorder.

Education and support are important for both patients and caregivers, and many communities offer such groups. Some groups deal specifically with issues related to Parkinson's disease, while in smaller communities support groups may attempt to address problems stemming from a mix of neurological conditions. Information about such groups in your community can be obtained from your neurologist, psychologist, primary doctor, or from sources such as the Internet. The National Parkinson Foundation has a website at NPF.org. The Neurology Research and Education Center of the Covenant Health System in Lubbock can be found at www.nrec.com.

Exercise and adequate nutrition are also important in maintaining mental functioning. Therapy programs have been developed specifically for Parkinson's disease patients, and these are discussed elsewhere in this book (see chapter 6, "Nursing Aspects of Parkinson's Disease," and chapter 7, "Occupational and Physical Therapy").

NEUROREHABILITATION

In addition, speech and cognitive rehabilitation therapies can help many patients develop strategies to circumvent some of their cognitive and memory limitations. Such services are available from licensed speech/ language pathologists and clinical neuropsychologists or geropsychologists.

Speech therapists can help the Parkinson's disease patient to speak more forcefully in order to be understood. They can also help the patient to overcome mild memory problems by training him or her in the use of various strategies and methods to become more independent regarding information that needs to be remembered. This type of therapy overlaps with cognitive rehabilitation programs that often are operated in neuropsychology clinics. Therapists in these programs use the results of neuropsychological tests to pinpoint the specific areas of change or weakness contributing to a patient's difficulties at home or at work. By providing practice at basic skills and development of strategies or compensatory devices designed for a particular patient's needs, they can help a patient either to rebuild his or her strength in a particular area of functioning, or to learn new ways to deal with specific types of information that are causing the patient difficulties.

SUGGESTED READINGS

Chui, H. C., Mortimer, J. A., Slager, V., Zarrow, C., Bondareff, W., and Webster, D. D. (1986). "Pathological correlates of dementia in Parkinson's disease." *Archives of Neurology* 43:991–95.

Elias, M. F., Elias, J. W., and Elias, P. K. (1988). "Biological and health influences on aging." In J. E. Birren and K. W. Schaie, eds., *Handbook of the Psychology of Aging.* New York: Academic Press.

Elias, M. F., Elias, J. W., and Elias, P. K. (1977). *Basic Processes in Adult Developmental Psychology.* St. Louis: Mosby.

Fisher, A., Hanin, I., and Lachman, C. (1986). *Alzheimer's and Parkinson's Disease: Strategies for Research and Development.* New York: Plenum Press.

Huber, S. J., Shuttleworth, E. C., and Paulson, G. W. (1986). "Dementia in Parkinson's disease." *Archives of Neurology* 43:987–90.

Mann, D. (1983). "The locus of coerulus and its possible role in aging and degenerative disease of the human central nervous system." *Mechanisms of Aging and Development* 23:73–79.

Mann, D. M., and Yates, P. O. (1982). "Pathogenesis of Parkinson's disease." *Archives of Neurology* 39:545–49.

Nauta, W., and Freitag, M. (1986). *Fundamental Neuroanatomy.* New York: Freeman and Co.

Whitehouse, P. J., Hedreen, J. C., White, C. L., and Price, D. L. (1983). "Basal forebrain neurons in the dementia of Parkinson's disease." *Annals of Neurology* 13:243–48.

14

Community Support Systems
Susan C. Imke

The purpose of this chapter is to suggest ways in which people with Parkinson's disease (PD) and their families may identify and access services from health care professionals, community agencies, and national organizations. Timely connections with such resources can help reduce feelings of apprehension and isolation.

HEALTH CARE PROFESSIONALS

Once a diagnosis of Parkinson's disease is made and a family begins the process of adjustment to living with a chronic disease, many people experience a "Where do I turn?" response. It is reasonable to begin the quest for knowledge by seeking information from the physician who confirmed the diagnosis of PD. The doctor or another health care professional on the medical team should be able to address specific questions in depth and suggest additional resources.

It is wise to seek out physicians to supervise your medical care that are knowledgeable about Parkinson's disease. At minimum, this medical team should include a neurologist (preferably a movement disorders specialist) and a primary care physician, usually a family practitioner or internist. Licensed physicians in the U.S. hold either an M.D. (doctor of medicine) or a D.O. (doctor of osteopathy) credential, and are often assisted by nurse practitioners, physician assistants, or other health care professionals who are qualified to provide information and advice to families regarding PD.

EDUCATIONAL LITERATURE

An array of basic as well as advanced patient education publications are available to assist individuals and families in learning more about the disease and strategies for making necessary lifestyle adaptations. Oftentimes, a person just diagnosed with Parkinson's disease is emotionally overwhelmed and may over-react to or misinterpret information if the content is too voluminous or complicated.

Once such an individual has had time to "absorb" the diagnosis and understand initial treatment options, then s/he is more likely to be receptive to and helped by receiving more detailed information. The National Parkinson Foundation has a new series of educational manuals that are excellent resources for learning more about the disease process, prognosis, and encouraging news about treatments and research.

SUPPORT GROUP INTERVENTIONS

Parkinson's disease support groups provide a "common plight" forum through which families can share their expertise and concerns. Support groups are often sponsored by voluntary health agencies such as the National Parkinson Foundation or the American Parkinson Disease Association. Biweekly or monthly meetings typically focus on a program, speaker, or discussion topic targeted to families who want to learn more about the disease and offer encouragement and support to one another.

Sometimes patients or physicians express concern that attending such gatherings might be discouraging or depressing. On the contrary, recently diagnosed patients typically have an opportunity to visit with numerous people who have had the disease for many years and are managing quite well. Regular participants often identify the support group experience as a valued aspect of their lives. A newcomer is likely to feel *encouraged* and uplifted following the initial contact with such a group. Empathetic concern from someone who's "been there" can be very reassuring that life with PD will continue to be productive and have meaning.

In addition to camaraderie and education, some groups also sponsor ancillary services to aid both patients and care partners. These may include exercise groups, speech therapy sessions, shared transportation to meetings, separate discussion groups for spouses, and equipment loan "closets."

COMMUNITY SERVICES

Community social-service agencies provide a variety of services for senior adults that can be helpful to persons with PD whose goal is to continue to manage independent living. The federal government provides funding to Area Agencies on Aging (AAA) in most U.S. cities and towns. AAA funds senior centers which serve the population over age 60 and offer social, educational, and health-maintenance programs in addition to midday meal service. Many senior centers also work with Meals on Wheels or other programs to provide a hot lunch to homebound seniors.

Some AAA senior centers provide transportation to the center, medical appointments, and other essential errands for persons who qualify. Transportation varies from scheduled routes in larger cities to demand/response in smaller communities.

One of the most frustrating losses a person can experience is the ability to drive safely. As the disease progresses, physicians or family members may recommend that a person with PD discontinue driving. If a spouse or other caregiver is willing and able to take the wheel, this loss may be mostly an inconvenience. But for the disabled individual who lives alone, being unable to drive constitutes a major handicap. Utilization of the AAA transportation services can help prevent social isolation.

Other services offered by Area Agencies on Aging include:

- *Information and referral* to assist in obtaining help with such matters as Social Security and Medicare benefits, employment and educational opportunities, health-care services, legal aid, volunteer opportunities, and shared housing programs.
- *Adult day care* to access nonresidential day activity centers, which provide weekday care to individuals who cannot safely stay alone but do not require skilled nursing care. Day activity centers are an affordable option to in-home care and offer much-needed respite to family caregivers. In some cases, the availability of quality day care for elders provides caregivers the opportunity to continue gainful employment.
- *Legal assistance* to counsel families regarding the preparation of a will, establishing a power of attorney, signing advanced directives, making property decisions, reporting consumer fraud, and understanding one's legal rights.
- *Case management* to provide an ombudsman to coordinate with community resources to help with complicated or multiple prob-

lems such as poor health, fixed income, lack of health insurance, inadequate housing, elder abuse, etc.

INTERMEDIATE CARE OPTIONS

Licensed home health agencies and foster-care group homes are additional resources in most communities for people with Parkinson's disease who need care beyond what family and friends can provide. Need for this level of service may be permanent, relative to the progression of the disease and subsequent degree of impairment, or may be short term, following an acute illness, injury, or hospitalization.

While Medicare may cover partial expenses for these services when ordered by a physician, Medicare guidelines and restrictions are under constant scrutiny and revision; a family considering home health or foster-care options should always inquire, *in advance of contracting for service*, to what extent the desired service will be covered or reimbursed by their health insurance provider(s).

Home health services can include initial need assessment by a registered nurse, social work consultation, physical and occupational therapy, speech therapy, and other services which vary from one agency and community to another. Agency personnel can recommend and make arrangements to acquire medical equipment which can greatly simplify physical care at home.

RESIDENTIAL CARE

It is estimated that only 15 to 20 percent of persons with Parkinson's disease will ever require extended nursing home care. Nevertheless, it behooves family caregivers to know how to recognize quality in a skilled nursing care facility should the need arise. Despite a trend toward progressive level-of-care retirement communities and group foster homes for those who can no longer live in their own homes, most people who require residential care still utilize the services of traditional nursing homes.

The following criteria are intended to serve as guidelines to help families identify reputable long-term care centers:

- The facility, administrator, and the director of nursing services should have current licenses from the state. Request an appointment with the administrator and the director of nursing to discuss the needs of your relative as a prospective resident. Inquire about their knowledge of PD and experience caring for patients with Parkinson's disease.

- Ideally, the facility should have a registered nurse on duty (versus on call) 24 hours per day.
- Cleanliness is a good indicator of the overall quality of care. Inspect the kitchen and bathroom areas. Bits of food on the dining-room floor during mealtimes is understandable, but should be promptly cleaned afterwards. Since incontinence is a problem for many nursing home residents, a faint odor of urine early in the morning is inevitable. However, any strong or persistent odor of urine or feces throughout the day should caution a family away from that facility.
- Observe the condition of clothing and grooming of residents. Disarrayed or soiled clothing can be a clue to poor nursing standards or understaffing.
- Visit the facility unannounced, at different times of the day and evening. Observe whether nursing staff responds promptly to patient call lights and other requests for help. What is their manner and attitude in talking with patients?
- The physical plant should be pleasant and relatively quiet. People with movement disorders need wide hallways with handrails along the walls. Bathrooms must be accessible for wheelchairs. Families deserve a visiting place away from roommates and communal dining areas.
- If your loved one with Parkinson's disease also has dementia (confusion), inquire if the staff is adequately trained to cope with and assist patients with cognitive problems.
- Inquire about patient-to-staff ratios and personnel turnover rates. The best care facilities have nurses and aides who genuinely enjoy working with older adults. Determine if the physician who now manages the care of your relative will continue to do so in the nursing home, or decide if you will feel comfortable with the medical director of the facility overseeing that care.

Many patients and family members dread having to make the nursing home decision. The reality for many families is that the experience is more positive than imagined. Primary family caregivers can remain involved in the care of their spouses or parents by providing outings on weekends or holidays, spending time in the loved one's "new home," and retaining the role of care supervisor—ensuring that the level of care received in the facility remains high. It is truly possible for families and nursing home staff members to collaborate to meet the special needs of persons with advanced Parkinson's disease.

NATIONAL ORGANIZATIONS

Voluntary health organizations such as the National Parkinson Foundation (NPF) and the American Parkinson Disease Association (APDA) sponsor regional networks that offer a variety of services to families living with Parkinson's disease. These include referrals to neurologists who specialize in the diagnosis and treatment of Parkinson's disease. There are currently 40 NPF Centers of Excellence in the U.S. and Canada that provide medical services, research updates, and educational services. These range from providing extensive educational literature free of charge to hosting regional seminars for patients and families who wish to obtain the latest information about PD and health maintenance.

Other national organizations such as the American Red Cross and the American Heart Association provide valuable services to families living with PD, such as training in cardiopulmonary resuscitation (CPR) and the Heimlich maneuver to rescue someone who is choking. Since some persons with advanced Parkinson's disease have swallowing problems and are at risk for airway obstruction due to choking, caregivers are advised to learn these simple and potentially life-saving techniques.

TIPS FOR TRAVELING

It is not uncommon for families faced with living with a progressive chronic illness to decide to take advantage of opportunities to travel while health and energy levels will allow them to fully enjoy the leisure activities and new destinations.

Many options exist to make the travel experience safe and comfortable. For instance, an individual who may not require the use of any mobility aids in his home environment might do well to reserve a wheelchair to navigate long airport corridors and busy terminals. A travel agent can arrange in advance for escort and/or wheelchair services from the baggage check point to the gate. Other than minimal gratuities, there is no charge for this service.

For people who do not need or choose to use wheelchair services, rented luggage strollers, available in many U.S. airports under the trade name Smarte Carte, are an inexpensive vehicle not only to transport luggage, but to steady one's balance in much the same manner as walking behind a grocery cart. A simple walking cane can be used to "point balance" through crowded passageways, and also carries a subtle message that an altered gait or balance problem is due to a health condition and not intoxication!

The cardinal travel tip for persons with Parkinson's disease is to keep PD medications with you at all times. It is also wise to pack extra doses of medications with you in the event that atypical eating patterns and activity levels result in a temporary need for extra dopamine replacement therapy.

Packing lighter and limiting carry-on baggage greatly simplifies air travel. Lost luggage on nonstop and direct flights is actually a very rare occurrence.

The following additional travel tips are taken from the web site "Awakenings" (contact information provided at the end of this chapter):

- When possible, travel with a relative or friend. Carry some identification that says you have PD. (Cards are available from the National Parkinson Foundation.)
- Take along a small bottle of water and invest in a collapsible cup to ensure that medication doses can be taken on time with a minimum of hassle.
- Wear your most comfortable clothes and shoes. Ill-fitting shoes can ruin the most carefully planned vacation! Wear a "fanny pack" rather than carrying a purse; having both hands free greatly improves balance.
- *Pace yourself.* Limiting major activities or outings to one or two events per day will avoid exhaustion and temporarily increasing the severity of Parkinson symptoms.
- Ask your travel agent to check ahead on hotel accommodations for disabled persons. Request being placed on the ground floor or near an elevator. Pack a nightlight to avoid falls in dark hotel rooms.

Cruise ship travel is often a relaxed way to travel in lieu of frequent hotel changes and luggage handling. Ship crews are accustomed to travelers with special needs and often go out of their way to be helpful.

Consider vacation destinations that are closer to home. A good guideline is to choose flights shorter than three hours. Exotic foreign destinations have their allure, but often the easier trip turns out to be the best trip! Car travel affords the luxury of determining the itinerary, daily agenda, and bathroom and snack breaks at the convenience or need of the person with PD, as opposed to hectic airline and group tour schedules. Investigate nearby cities or resorts that you've never had time to explore and do so at your own pace.

CLOSER TO HOME

Handicapped parking permits simplify local and long-distance travel for people with impaired mobility. Applications forms can be obtained through state motor vehicle agencies or local county or parish clerk offices. These must be signed by a licensed physician certifying the handicap.

The card can be placed on the dashboard of any vehicle occupied by the person with a disability. Using such a permit enables many persons with PD to shop and take care of business independently.

Finally, it is important to remember that community support is a two-way street. This chapter has focused on helping people with Parkinson's disease to access vital support services in the communities in which they live. It is equally important for them to remain active contributors *to* those communities.

Whether you live in a city or a small town, local support groups, churches, charities, and civic groups need mature volunteers to devote time and energy to ongoing projects. People with PD can positively influence their communities in many ways—from serving on city council committees to organizing public awareness about Parkinson's disease.

Continued engagement in meaningful life pursuits is good preventive medicine to guard against chronic discouragement, self-absorption, mental atrophy, and premature physical decline. Families living with Parkinson's disease can learn to accept help in meeting their own needs while simultaneously sharing their unique experience with others.

RESOURCES

• **National Parkinson Foundation, Inc.**
 1501 N.W. 9th Avenue
 Miami, Florida 33136-1494

 Phone: (800) 327-4545 or (305) 547-6666
 Fax: (305) 243-4403
 Web Site: http://www.parkinson.org

- **Outreach Programs**—comprehensive outpatient rehabilitation services, including physical therapy, occupational therapy, and speech therapy, at a variety of sites in the U.S.

  Phone: (800) 243-3333

- **Awakenings** Web Site: http://www.parkinsonsdisease.com

- **Parkinson's Digest** Web Site: http://www.harfordweb.com/pd/

- **Muhammad Ali Parkinson Research Center**
  Barrow Neurological Institute
  Phoenix, Arizona

  Phone: (602) 406-4931
  Fax: (602) 406-6131

15

Caregivers Need Care, Too

Trudy Hutton

Margaret Mead, the noted anthropologist, said that "societies are judged by how they care for the most vulnerable among them: the elderly, the poor, the mentally ill." Who are the people giving this care, and who takes care of the caregivers?

It has been estimated that only 10 percent to 20 percent of people needing care in this country receive it in institutions. The remaining 80 to 90 percent are cared for at home by family caregivers, usually a spouse or child. Family caregivers provide assistance ranging from an hour of grocery shopping or a daily phone call to total, round-the-clock care for a house-bound or bedridden loved one. The majority of care is usually provided by one person in the family. Most caregivers—an estimated 80 percent—are women.

Caregiving is an important role requiring patience, commitment, and dedication. It can also be a very stressful role, exhausting the caregiver physically and emotionally. At some point in the caregiving process, most caregivers show the signs of chronic stress and strain. They feel over-whelmed and unrewarded. The caregiver lacks energy for relating to friends and family. Sometimes referred to as "compassion fatigue," this psychological state leaves the caregiver feeling depleted, numb, and exhausted. Unlike normal fatigue, compassion fatigue is not alleviated by a good night's rest. Too often the caregiver is unable to see the signs of distress or is unwilling to seek assistance. Left unattended, compassion fatigue can lead to deeper problems of burnout, physical illness, or clinical depression. It is of the utmost importance that caregivers take time out to care for themselves.

Primary caregivers run a high risk of neglecting themselves mentally, spiritually, and physically. Caregiving requires a major change in the life of the caregiver as well as the life of the patient. Caregiving keeps the caregiver off balance psychologically and physically. It is easy for the caregiver to enter into a downward spiral of sadness, frustration, stress, and strain on both the body and the mind. Simple everyday tasks such as running to the store or taking a spontaneous walk may become logistically challenging. Routine tasks may become difficult or virtually impossible.

Most caregivers think they should or must personally provide all of the care for their loved one. They work day and night to compensate for the changes that Parkinson's disease has made in their lives and the lives of their loved one. Caregiving may become a personal challenge in which the caregiver seeks to prove herself as the perfect wife or daughter. The caregiver may refuse help and yet stay up all night doing laundry. He or she may not discuss the Parkinson's disease with family and friends, and yet feel as if he or she is in it all alone. A caregiver may make social plans and become frustrated when the Parkinson's disease prevents following them through. Such unrealistic expectations are a sure route to physical, mental, and emotional exhaustion.

Because the primary caregiver is often solely responsible for the majority of care for the patient, you must consider what will happen to the patient should you have some serious physical or emotional crisis that results in your inability to provide care. All too often, no one else is available to step into the caregiver's role. It is, therefore, of utmost importance that as the caregiver you also take care of yourself. The familiar safety message given on airplanes during takeoff has been cited as comparable. You are told how to buckle your seat belt and how to use the seat cushion as a flotation device. You are told what to do if the cabin loses pressure and oxygen masks drop down. "If you are traveling with a small child or someone who needs extra assistance, secure your own mask first . . ." The message is that you cannot help someone else if you are gasping for air yourself. You cannot give and give without renewing your own energy or eventually you will give out. If your health—mental or physical—is not maintained, both you and your patient will suffer. It is important to step out of the caregiver role on a regular basis and rekindle your spirit. Learn to give to yourself in addition to giving to others.

EMOTIONAL DILEMMAS
OF CAREGIVERS

When a family member is diagnosed with a chronic illness, the whole family is affected. Parkinson's disease is no different. It effects unexpected changes in the lifestyle of patient, spouse, children, and perhaps parents or siblings. You are all partners in Parkinson's disease. In most cases, the transition into caregiving is sudden. You find yourself in a job for which you did not ask and for which you have not been trained. A whole range of feelings and emotions confront the caregiver. You feel a sadness and sense of loss that you cannot do the things you and your loved one had planned. You are frightened by what the future may hold and perhaps by the new responsibilities thrust upon you. Anxiety and a feeling of helplessness emerge. Financial repercussions may develop. You may feel uncomfortable or humiliated to have to ask for help from others. Caregiving produces an emotional roller coaster for which the caregiver is not prepared.

Caregiving challenges you to cultivate your own inner strength so that you can meet the needs of your loved one and at the same time maintain your own well-being. Be prepared for a wide range of feelings that you might consider negative, such as guilt, anger, and jealousy.

Guilt is one of the most common emotions experienced by caregivers. You may feel that you are not doing enough to help your loved one, even though you are "at the end of your rope." You may feel trapped, resentful, angry, and burdened. You may feel sorry for yourself for being robbed of your plans for the future. You may believe you are doing a thankless job and are not appreciated. Then you feel guilty about this resentment and anger because you are not the one with the disease. You may feel guilty for not being able to control the disease or the impact it has on you and your loved one. If you feel your life is spinning out of control, take charge of what you can control. Pay attention to times when you feel as if you have done all you can. Ask yourself if there is anything more you can do. Then allow yourself the peace of mind that comes from having done your best.

You may find yourself resentful and angry. You may resent the way the illness has altered your life or your loved one's dependence on you. You may feel isolated from family and friends. You may be surprised to discover that your loved one is as angry and frustrated as you are. Anger and resentment are normal; just be sure that you direct the anger and resentment at the illness and not at your loved one, or at others who try to help you. Find healthy ways to vent your anger. Get in the car, turn up the radio, and scream as loud as you can. Try pounding nails or beating the bed with a tennis racket or broom. Exercise is a good way to vent anger and strengthen you physically at the same time. Meditation or relaxation techniques may work for you. Find a friend and confidant or counselor to whom you can confide your feelings. Don't let anger seethe. To do so is physically draining as well as emotionally depleting.

You may feel jealous of the attention that your loved one receives and think that no one is concerned about your well-being. You find that friends and family identify with the patient and ask about his or her well-being. You may feel invisible and ignored. Nobody asks how you are coping or how your health is or if you are eating well. You are lonely and need a shoulder to cry on, but nobody asks about your needs.

We often think of the grief process as coming into play at the death of a loved one, but grief is a normal emotion for any loss. When you become a caregiver to someone with a chronic illness, you find yourself faced with a number of losses in your life. Losses may range from your weekly bridge game to a loss of freedom and privacy. List the losses you experience, even those you might consider small losses, and give yourself permission to grieve these losses. Be patient with yourself through the grieving process. A good cry is a valuable way to release pain, anger, frustration, and grief.

Guilt, anger, jealousy, and grief are among the normal and expected reactions in a caregiving situation. Emotions are real and deserve your attention. It is important to identify your emotions so that you can better understand them and how they affect you. The feelings you experience may not make sense to you, but remember that feelings are neither right nor wrong. The key is how you deal with them. To do your best as a caregiver, it is important to acknowledge your emotions, even if it is just to yourself. Once they have been identified, you can confront them and learn how to deal with them.

Learning to live with your feelings is easier if you let others help. Find someone you can talk to about your feelings, someone who can help you regain a positive perspective. It may be another caregiver, a close friend, or a professional counselor. Surround yourself with people whom you love and who can help you appreciate the strengths and talents you possess. You may become more compassionate and patient; you may develop a greater appreciation for what you still have. You may find you have an inner strength you did not know you possessed. It is helpful to recognize that you may have grown from the caregiving experience.

STRESS

Caregiving can be very satisfying as an expression of love and caring for someone important in your life. It also creates stresses that can be physically and emotionally draining. Stress from caregiving varies from day to day depending upon the responsibilities which arise, your loved one's circumstances, and your own health and energy level. Stress tends to increase if circumstances become more uncontrollable and uncertain. Some stressors most caregivers face include:

- Taking on new financial or household responsibilities

- Managing health care for another individual

- Becoming the sole means of transportation or companionship

- Lack of sleep.

Stressors include not only the general demands and responsibilities of caregiving, but also adjustments to changing roles and losses you have experienced. Managing stress is a balancing act which requires balancing the demands of your life with the resources available to help you cope with these demands.

At times stress can build up before the caregiver realizes it, compassion fatigue sets in, and then you are in danger of suffering burnout. Burnout happens gradually and in stages. Burnout affects the health, motivation, and attitude of the caregiver and can spill over into other aspects of life. It is important to learn to recognize the warning signs of stress and anticipate the situations which create or increase stress for you. Once you recognize and anticipate stressors, you can take the time to relieve them before they reach a critical stage. You probably cannot eliminate all stress in your life, but you can learn to control and reduce it before you reach the compassion fatigue or burnout stage. Some warning signs of stress include:

- Feeling a loss of energy or zest for life

- Feeling out of control

- Lacking a time or place to be alone

- Feeling overwhelmed economically, emotionally, or physically

- Exhibiting uncharacteristic emotions or actions

- Lacking interest in people or things that were formerly pleasurable

- Becoming increasingly isolated

- Sleep problems (either too much or too little)

- Appetite changes

- Consuming increasing amounts of medications, alcohol, caffeine, or cigarettes

- Increasing health problems

- Problems with concentration or memory

- Increasing irritability or impatience with others

- Feeling angry with the person you care for

- Feeling it's selfish to think of yourself

- Thoughts of suicide.

Recognize what you can and cannot do about stressors and make the necessary accommodations in your life. Don't "should" yourself to death; learn to let go of things that really do not matter and focus on those things that do. It is not important that the dishes get washed after every meal or that the bed is made every day. It may be more important for your own well-being to take a few minutes for a walk in the garden or some other relaxing activity, or to enjoy some special time with your loved one or friends. When things get rough, take a break. Even the bathroom provides a few minutes of quiet and privacy.

Some stress relievers include washing a car, digging in the garden, taking a brisk walk, listening to favorite music, or performing relaxation exercises. Learn what works for you and utilize those methods when you feel stress building up.

TAKING CARE OF YOURSELF

In addition to coping with your emotions and stress, a number of things can be done as a caregiver to maintain your own sense of well-being. It is important to look after yourself in order to be a good caregiver. What works for one caregiver may not work for another. Solutions are as unique as each caregiver and patient. Consider these suggestions, which apply in most situations and which will help you be the best caregiver you can while maintaining your own dignity and sense of self worth:

Educate yourself. Information is among the top ten needs of caregivers; information about the disease and about caregiving responsibilities enables you to cope successfully with the illness. Learn as much as you can: Locate books, pamphlets, videotapes, and news articles on Parkinson's disease, medications, treatment, and research. This not only helps you understand the disease process and what you might expect in the future, it also helps you formulate knowledgeable questions for your visits to your physician. The National Parkinson Foundation Centers of Excellence are good resources for literature and videotapes. Your local libraries may have current books about Parkinson's disease as well as books about caregiving and other types of information you might find useful, from financial planning to exercise techniques. Libraries also have lists of community resources which may be available to you. If you have access to the Internet, a number of web sites are devoted to Parkinson's disease and caregiving which not only provide information about the disease, but also connections to others who are dealing with Parkinson's challenges. A word of caution, however, about Internet sites: The information which appears on the Internet is not regulated and ranges from excellent to questionable.

Find a Parkinson's disease support group for both of you where you can express fears and emotions you may not yet be able to express to each other at home. Good support groups provide emotional support, practical knowledge, and assistance for both patient and caregiver. Support groups give both partners an opportunity to meet and share with others who face the same challenges of dealing with the disease. Support group members represent a broad range of experiences dealing with all stages of Parkinson's disease. There are few problems you might face that have not already been dealt with by some member of the group. Support groups also provide a comfortable social situation in which the patient and caregiver can relax and feel accepted. To locate a support group, ask your physician or nurse or contact the National Parkinson Foundation for support groups in your area.

Be kind to yourself. Nurture your self-esteem. Self-esteem is vital to your well-being and your ability to cope with stress. Pay attention to what you say to yourself and watch for self-critical statements. Replace your negative thoughts with reasonable and positive ones which acknowledge your situation and recognize your strengths and abilities. Spend time with your "fan club," people who help you believe in yourself and recognize your capabilities. Know your limits of time, energy, and capabilities and keep your self-expectations realistic. Anticipate your needs and cut back or set limits on the demands on your energy and time. Setting limits may be hard, but ultimately it proves to be self-destructive not to do so. Learn to say no.

Maintain your own health. Your own health affects not only your ability to cope with caregiving but also your outlook on life. If you allow your own health to deteriorate, the care you are able to provide for your loved one will also deteriorate. If you suffer a health crisis, who will take care of your loved one? Make and keep appointments with your doctor for routine check-ups as well as for medical care for your own health problems. If you take prescription medication, be as diligent about taking your medicine as you are about your loved one's taking his medicine. Develop a healthy life style for yourself.

Exercise for 20 minutes or more a day at least three times a week. Regular exercise will help you keep in shape, sleep better, and have more energy. Exercise promotes relaxation and reduces stress. It also improves balance, coordination, and mood. Forego excuses for not exercising such as being too old, not having enough time, or getting enough exercise from your daily routine of caregiving. Exercise can be tailored to the needs, abilities, and time constraints of the individual.

Choose an exercise you enjoy, benefit from, and will continue doing. The more you enjoy an exercise program, the better the chance you will stick to it. It is more likely that you will continue your exercise program if someone else participates with you. Find a friend and begin an exercise routine together. Another option is to join an exercise class. This not only provides an incentive to stay on the exercise program, it gives one companions for support and encouragement. Check with local hospitals, the YMCA, the YWCA, and fitness centers for available exercise classes at your ability level. There are several good exercise books and videotapes available from bookstores or libraries.

Don't expect too much too soon. The results of your exercise program will be greater if you set short-term goals and build up slowly. Begin by exercising regularly two or three times a week. Incorporate your exercise program into your regular routine and work up to including exercise in your schedule every day. Swimming, bicycling, golf, or tennis may be exercise options. Walking is an exercise available to you almost any-where and at any time. Even a brisk walk around the block can provide a break and refresh the spirit.

Regardless of the exercise method you choose to follow, you should obtain medical clearance from your physician. If you have any questions about specific exercises to include, a physical therapist or exercise trainer can help design a program which will be most beneficial for you.

Get enough rest. Your need for sleep varies with the demands of your life. Get enough sleep so that you wake up feeling rested and refreshed. If your nightly sleep is interrupted, take a nap during the day. If your care-giving demands make sleep difficult during the day, find someone who can replace you for a couple of hours so that you can rest. If you can afford extra help, hire someone to provide daytime relief. If you cannot afford to hire someone, ask a friend or relative if they can relieve you during the day. Support group members are also a source of assistance.

You may find falling asleep difficult if you are tense or too exhausted. Learn some relaxation techniques which work for you. Deep-breathing exercises, meditation, and biofeedback are some methods available to help you relax. A number of books, audio tapes, and videotapes describing relaxation techniques are available from bookstores and libraries. Community centers, hospitals, YMCAs, and YWCAs frequently offer relaxation classes. Ask your health care provider or counselor for recommendations for relaxation methods or programs.

Eat well. Too often caregivers overlook the basic need of eating a balanced diet themselves. They are concerned that their loved one gets a proper diet and eats sufficiently to maintain his health. Yet too often, after preparing a meal for the loved one, perhaps helping him eat, and then cleaning up, a caregiver is too tired or tense to pay attention to her own diet. It is easy to fall into the "cereal and milk" habit, eating a snack on the run, or eating over the kitchen sink.

A healthy diet consists of a variety of foods every day from the main food groups: bread, the cereal and pasta group, the fruit and vegetable group, the meat group, and the dairy group. Limit your intake of salt and highly salted foods. Eat foods low in saturated fat and cholesterol, and avoid too much red meat, fried foods, and rich desserts. Include fiber in your diet by eating a lot of fresh fruits, vegetables, and cereals. Maintain your weight; don't gain or lose pounds. Limit sweets and caffeine. Too much coffee or sugar could put you on edge and make your caregiving duties more difficult.

In addition to maintaining a healthy diet, the caregiver should provide herself a pleasant mealtime atmosphere. If you and your loved one can eat together, make mealtime a pleasant time to talk to one another. If you eat alone, put on music you enjoy, get out the good china, and take the time to enjoy your meal. Move to a window or a porch where you can enjoy a view while you eat. Invite friends to join you (or you and your loved one) for a meal. Making mealtime a pleasant experience improves your chances of maintaining a balanced diet and sound eating habits.

Give yourself a break. Because so much of your caregiving abilities depends on emotional well-being, it is especially important that a caregiver set aside some time every day as personal time. It is not selfish to take care of yourself or to take time for yourself. It is a way of honoring and valuing human life and your own value as a human being. While you may need a break from caregiving, your loved one may also need a break from you. Getting away from your caregiving responsibilities may not eliminate the problems you face, but it can make you feel better and give you energy to face a new day.

Get out of the house as much as you can. If you find it difficult to get away from the house, a simple change of scene is helpful. Get some fresh air by taking a walk in your yard, sitting on the porch, or watching the stars come out. Use the telephone as a support line when you can't get away.

Personal time may be only 15 or 20 minutes a day, but taking some time out consistently every day is more important that the amount of time taken. Do something you enjoy with your personal time: take a walk, listen to music, read a book, garden, go fishing. Practice skills for which you receive affirmation. Maintain your hobbies. Don't give up activities that keep you "plugged in" to life. Try something new. Activities that refresh your mind and spirit are an important part of coping with the stresses of caregiving.

At least once a week, plan an enjoyable activity for yourself away from home. Have lunch with a friend or get your hair done. Attend seminars and classes that promote personal or professional growth. Use personal time to enrich your life and to keep your mind active. Running necessary errands, grocery shopping, and doctors' appointments do not count as personal time.

Be social. Make it a priority to maintain contact with friends and family. If you find yourself becoming isolated from family and friends, make an effort to renew old ties and develop new ones. Use the telephone to maintain contact with friends and connections with family. Go to worship services, help a neighbor, participate in volunteer work. Stay involved with people. Don't let your caregiving responsibilities tie you down or cut you off from social contact. Look at the long-term picture. If you cut all social ties and devote yourself to caregiving to the exclusion of everything else, you will find in the long term you have given and given and have nothing left.

It may not be easy to take time away from your caregiving activities, especially if your loved one protests. It is up to you, however, to plan for your personal time and pursue your own interests. Remember that a few hours or a few days away will make your a better caregiver.

Set realistic goals and change unrealistic expectations. Caregiving is probably one of many demands on your time and energy. Evaluate your expectations regularly to eliminate idealized expectations, such as always knowing what your loved one wants or how he feels or always being patient and supportive. Let go of these idealized expectations and set reasonable goals. It is not important that the house is vacuumed or the laundry done every day. It may be more important that you and your loved one enjoy some quality time together, or that you get an extra nap to catch up on missed sleep. Bolster independence in your loved one. Encourage him to do as much as he can for himself, even if it takes longer to get done. Prioritize your responsibilities and act accordingly. Recognize what you can and cannot do as well as what really needs to be done. Find ways of getting things done without doing all of them yourself. No one can "do it all."

Let others help. When someone offers to help, consider it a sincere offer and accept it. When people are tired of helping, they will stop offering. Regard it as a gift to them to be able to do something for another. Make an inventory of what you need done and write it down. When someone asks if there is anything they can do, consult the list. Perhaps you might give the volunteer a choice of things you need done: pick up a prescription, do grocery shopping, or clean gutters. Maybe you can exchange services with another caregiver. If you are buying groceries, you can pick up what a friend needs. When she is running an errand, she can pick up something for you. You might also consider exchanging meals so each of you cooks only half as often. Work with doctors, nurses, social workers, and clergy to identify other support resources in your community. Look for services through your local information and referral center, social service agencies, religious organizations, and county and city agencies. Many times you will find help with transportation, meals, household chores, and general help through these sources.

If no one volunteers, ask for the help you need. Many times friends and family members are willing to help, but if you appear to be coping well they may think you don't need help. Get your family together and explain your needs. Tell them, "I can do this, but I need you to do that." Sometimes family brainstorming sessions may create a unique solution you had not considered on your own. Build a caregiving team. Identify people you can count on as your support resources. They may be family members, friends, or support group members. Consider the individual's abilities and match helpers to your needs. Don't expect people to give what they can't. Finally, hiring help for some tasks may be an option if you can afford it.

There will be times that you need help for more than running errands or help around the house. You will need assistance with the caregiving responsibilities themselves, or you will need respite care for your loved one that will allow you some time away. Caregivers are often reluctant to trust actual caregiving to others. You may feel that you are the only one who can sufficiently provide for your loved one's needs, or that you are neglecting your responsibilities by allowing someone else to relieve you. Leaving your loved one in the care of another has been likened to a mother leaving a newborn for the first time.

Consider asking a member of your caregiving team to come in and stay with your loved one for a few hours on a regular basis. Inquire about adult day activity centers with scheduled programs and socialization with peers. If your loved one does not require care, but only companionship, check with senior citizen centers for programs and activities. On occasion, hospitals and residential care homes provide short-stay options at their facilities. Check with your Area Agency on Aging for possibilities. Remember that you are a more effective caregiver when you are rested and that there will come a time when you will need some respite, for a few hours or even for several days.

Plan for the time when you may need this type of help. The best time to seek this support is now, not when you are emotionally and physically exhausted and both your health and your relationships are suffering. Finding additional care to allow you time away may be a challenge, but having it available allows you to be a better caregiver. Using community-based resources will often postpone institutionalization. Give your support system a chance to work. Learn to let go. Delegate some of your responsibilities and allow others to help. No one person can do it all.

Communicate with your family and friends as well as your loved one. Communication is a key factor in successful caregiving. Talk to your loved one with Parkinson's disease. Both of you are making adjustments to the continuing changes Parkinson's disease brings. Showing a strong front while you are agonizing on the inside might be misinterpreted as lack of caring or compassion. While it may be unwise to share all of your feelings, maintain as much open communication as possible so that you are not controlled by the illness. It is important to share your feelings and not shut each other out. Be sure to share the full range of emotions; while sharing sadness and fear is important, it is also important to enjoy pleasurable moments and share the joy together.

Keep your family and friends informed about the disease in general and about how you and your patient are doing. Sharing thoughts and feelings is an important way to stay in touch and avoid feeling isolated. Sometimes relatives and friends can be critical about the way you provide care, how clean the house is, or how your loved one is dressed. They are responding to what they see without the benefit of the experience of day-to-day caregiving that you have. They may also be responding out of their own guilt about not participating more in the caregiving process.

Keeping them informed about the disease itself, about how you and your loved one are doing, about reports from the doctor, and about new research and scientific advances in Parkinson's disease will help them understand your situation better, as well as what they might expect as a result of the disease. Family conferences from time to time not only help other family members understand the situation but also involve them in the caregiving process. Set an agenda beforehand and don't try to cover too much at one meeting. Don't discuss extraneous complaints or ancient disagreements. If family members do criticize your caregiving, try to listen politely and acknowledge you have heard their concerns, even though it may be difficult. They may express some valid concern that you can address once you know what it is. They may suggest a solution to a problem that you have not considered. The bottom line, however, regardless of what others say, is that if you and your loved one are comfortable with the way you are providing care, then continue with what you are doing.

Laugh. Keep laughter in your life and maintain your sense of humor. Look at the lighter side or the ridiculous aspects of Parkinson's disease. Try to see the humor in being a caregiver. Read funny books or jokes. Rent old movies and enjoy old-fashioned slapstick humor. Listen to tapes that make you laugh. Cut out cartoons and put them on the refrigerator where you can enjoy them. Share something humorous with your loved one, a friend, or a family member. Attend social gatherings where there is light-hearted fun and joy. Laughter is the best defense against the darker side of caregiving. Laughter really is the best medicine.

Good caregiving is based on common sense, life experiences, and understanding that care is needed for a specific situation. To be a good caregiver, you must appreciate your own efforts, draw strength from what you can do, and provide love, care, and dignity for your loved one. Keep yourself in good condition, both physically and emotionally, to allow you to provide the best care for your loved one. Every day think about at least one thing that you and others appreciate about *you*. Don't minimize what you do or what you offer to others. Finally, don't forget to give yourself a pat on the back for a job well done.

SUGGESTED READINGS

Carter, Rosalynn. (1994). *Helping Yourself Help Others*. New York: Times Books.

Cole, Harry A. (1991). *Helpmates: Support in Times of Critical Illness*. Louisville: Westminster/John Knox Press.

Karr, Katherine. (1992). *Taking Time for Me: How Caregivers Can Effectively Deal with Stress*. Amherst, N.Y.: Prometheus Books.

National Family Caregivers Association, Inc. (1996). *The Resourceful Caregiver*. St. Louis: Mosby-Yearbook, Inc.

Niebuhr, Sheryl, and Royse, Jane. (1989). *Take Care!* St. Paul: Wilder Foundation.

Parke-Davis, Inc. (1994). *Caring for the Caregiver*. Morris Plains, N.J.: Parke-Davis/Warner-Lambert Company.

Pirie, Inez. (1996). *Coping with Caregiving*. Amarillo, Tx.: Ruhl Press.

Sherman, James R. (1988). *Mainstay: For the Well Spouse of the Chronically Ill*. Boston: Little, Brown and Company.

Visiting Nurses Association of America. (1997). *Caregiver's Handbook*. New York: DK Publishing, Inc.

16

Research in Parkinson's Disease
William C. Koller

INTRODUCTION

There is an incredible amount of research being performed in the area of Parkinson's disease. Hopefully this article will convey something of the depth and the excitement involved in the research currently ongoing for this disease. Never at any other time in history has there been so many new discoveries and so many people involved in the research effort in Parkinson's disease. Both basic scientists and clinical neurologists are involved in this research. In the course of this article, I will discuss current research involving the causes of Parkinson's disease and new therapeutic interventions for it, including drugs and surgical treatment.

CAUSES OF PARKINSON'S DISEASE

Clearly the most important issue in research in Parkinson's disease is finding the cause of this disorder. Both genetics and environmental causes have been suggested. Most likely the cause of Parkinson's disease is related to some combination of genetic susceptibility and exposure to environmental toxins. It is not unusual for patients with Parkinson's disease to have a positive family history. It has been found that as many as 15 percent of Parkinson's patients have someone else with Parkinson's disease in their family tree. Furthermore, the occasional clustering of Parkinson's disease in families has been repeatedly reported over the past century. There are reports in rare families of Parkinson's disease following one generation after another. However, some of these families did not have what we would consider typical Parkinson's disease. A recent study of twins with Parkinson's disease found that identical twins and nonidentical twins have the same incidence of Parkinson's disease. This is evidence against a genetic basis for Parkinson's disease. However, in this study among twin pairs in which the onset of Parkinson's disease for the index twin was under age 60, a much higher concordance rate existed in the identical (or monozygotic) twins as compared to the nonidentical (or diozygotic) twins. Therefore, although the twin studies do not suggest a strong genetic factor, they are consistent with some mode of inheritance or genetic predisposition in the younger patient which has yet to be defined.

Several families have been reported in which Parkinson's disease is passed down from one generation to another. This is called *autosomal dominant inheritance,* which means the chance of getting the disease is one out of two. One large Italian-American family, the Conturse family, appears to have a relatively typical Parkinson's disease and has been studied in some detail by Dr. Roger Duvoisin at the Robert Wood Johnson Medical Center in New Jersey. From his study of the Conturse family, Dr. Duvoisin found genetic linkage to chromosome 4 (4Q 21-25). Shortly thereafter, Dr. Polmeropoulos and his colleagues at the National Institute of Health found that a mutation in a protein, alpha-synuclein, occurred in this family. Subsequently, researchers found three Greek families with hereditary Parkinson's disease who also had a similar genetic deficit. However, when this deficit in alpha-synuclein was looked at in other families with Parkinson's disease and in sporadically occurring Parkinson's disease, the protein was not found. Clearly, this mutation represents only a very small amount of Parkinson's disease. However, it was found that alpha-synuclein exists in the Lewy body, which is the pathological hallmark of Parkinson's disease. The Lewy body is an inclusion body found in dying neurons in the substantia nigra, the part of the brain that is damaged in Parkinson's disease. Therefore, it is possible that the alpha-synuclein deficit may lead to some basic knowledge to help us understand why neurons die. Clearly this is an exciting finding, one that will lead to more basic knowledge about Parkinson's disease. Indeed, we are in a new era of research involving the genetic investigation of Parkinson's disease. The implications of these findings will certainly increase our understanding of Parkinson's disease in the future.

The environment also plays some role in causing Parkinson's disease. A chemical, MPTP, has been found to induce the clinical syndrome identical to Parkinson's disease in humans. In animals, this chemical will destroy substantia nigra cells. The initial individuals studied were young drug addicts who took MPTP as a contaminate of their illicit drugs of abuse. The fact that a simple chemical like MPTP can cause clinical parkinsonism and selectively cause changes in the brain has raised the question of whether other chemicals in the environment could possibly do the same. However, to date, no such chemicals have been identified. Certain risk factors—such as living in a rural environment, drinking well water, and exposure to industrial pollutants—have been identified. Another interesting concept is that some patients may possess deficits in metabolizing certain chemicals. Therefore, exposure to these chemicals in these susceptible individuals could cause parkinsonism, where in the majority of other individuals these chemicals would be detoxified. One issue that must be addressed in our understanding of Parkinson's disease is the concept of individual susceptibility. Why do some patients develop Parkinson's disease while others with similar backgrounds and environmental exposures do not? Further investigations into genetic/environmental interaction will undoubtedly provide some of these answers.

Another major area of advance has been our increase of understanding at the basic science level of the mechanisms related to substantia nigra cell death. It appears that there is a cascade of events involved in generating injury to substantia nigra cells. Many deficits have been described, including mitochondrial damage, oxidative stress, and increased excitotoxicity. Chemicals are being developed that could interfere with these processes. Since it appears that there is a cascade of events that leads to nigral cell death, interfering at various levels could prevent these cells from dying. This is the concept of *neuroprotection*. Could we interfere with the mechanism of cell death, stop the cells from dying, and therefore slow the rate of clinical symptoms? Another interesting concept has been labeled *neurorescue*. For neuroprotection, we try to protect the cells from getting sick. The concept of neurorescue is that the cells are already sick but can be prevented from dying with intervention. Therefore these cells would be dysfunctional, but could be saved and restored to normal functioning. There are many drugs that have been shown in the laboratory to be capable of preventing cell death. The next challenge is to test these drugs to see if they are safe in animals and humans and then test to see if they are effective in slowing the rate of progression of Parkinson's disease. Unfortunately, there is no easy way to study the concepts of neuroprotection and neurorescue in patients with Parkinson's disease. However, some of these agents are being tested and hopefully within the next several years will be available to many more patients.

The concept of neuroprotection is a profound one. In my opinion, the next quantum leap in the treatment of Parkinson's disease will be the introduction of neuroprotective agents that are able to slow the rate of progression of the disease. Because it is estimated that 30 to 40 percent of cells die before the first symptom of Parkinson's disease is observed, early detection is important. There are several ongoing studies to see if Parkinson's disease can be detected before the patient exhibits clinical symptoms. These tests include the analysis of movement and reaction times, which can be slowed in early Parkinson's disease; testing the sense of smell, which is also deficient in early Parkinson's disease; and looking at various neuroimaging studies which can directly measure the dopamine system and detect dopamine loss in patients who have no symptoms.

Another major advance has been an increase in our understanding of the exact mechanism of how cells die in Parkinson's disease. It used to be thought that the process was *necrosis,* where cells basically disintegrated because of dysfunction. However, it appears that in Parkinson's disease and many other degenerative diseases, the process is one of apoptosis. *Apoptosis* refers to "cell suicide" or programmed cell death—that is, cells basically turn on mechanisms and commands that will result in their own destruction. Drugs have been studied in the laboratory that are anti-apototic and can interfere with this process. These drugs will also be studied in the not too distant future in Parkinson's disease patients to see if it is possible to halt the progression of the disease.

Clearly, there are many lines of investigation and many promising leads to help us understand the cause of Parkinson's disease and, more importantly, to have methods at our disposal that will block the mechanisms responsible for cell death in Parkinson's disease.

DRUG THERAPY

Drug therapy has been the mainstay for the treatment of Parkinson's disease. Many new agents are currently being tested, resulting in the clinician's arsenal for the treatment of Parkinson's disease being increased dramatically.

Levodopa

Levodopa remains the mainstay for the treatment of Parkinson's disease; however, complications such as dyskinesias and motor fluctuations compromise its long-term use. It was previously thought that about 40 to 50 percent of patients develop motor fluctuations after five years. In a recently published study, 618 patients were randomized either to Sinemet immediate release to Sinemet controlled release and followed for five years. The results of this study indicate that only about 20 percent of patients develop motor fluctuations and dyskinesia and that, for the most part, patients did well over the first five years of treatment with just levodopa-containing compounds. In addition, the dose of levodopa used in this study was relatively low: 425 mg for the immediate release Sinemet group and approximately 510 mg for the controlled release Sinemet group. This study is important because it indicates that levodopa-containing compounds can control Parkinson's disease well for the first five years of therapy with minimal complications.

Dopamine Agonists

Dopamine agonists are another class of drugs that are useful in the treatment of Parkinson's disease, both as early monotherapy and as adjuvants to levodopa therapy in more advanced disease. Two new dopamine agonists introduced into the market in 1998 are ropinerole and pramipexole. This brings the number of dopamine agonists available for the treatment of Parkinson's disease in the United States to four. This is important because the more drugs we have to treat Parkinson's disease—even drugs in a similar category—the more options we can offer the patient. Although these drugs have some similarities, it is clear that some patients respond better to one drug than to another or that one patient may have side effects from one but not another. It is interesting to note that dopomine agonists appear to be associated with less long-term complications than with levodopa; however, it is generally thought that these drugs do not control the symptoms of Parkinson's disease as well as levodopa. In younger patients, many clinicians now start with a dopamine agonist as their initial therapy and add levodopa at a later date. In the older patients, levodopa is often started first and dopamine agonists are added subsequently. The established concept now in the therapeutics of Parkinson's disease is combination therapy: using multiple drugs to obtain good control of symptoms, but with fewer side effects than in the past. Current research therefore indicates that the use of levodopa compounds and dopamine agonists together is very helpful in managing Parkinson's disease for the long term.

There is much interest from patients in skin patch therapy for the treatment of Parkinson's disease. Because of its physical and chemical characteristics, levadopa will never be able to be put into a patch. Other drugs are being studied in patch format, and one dopamine agonist in particular has been extensively studied in the patch format. This drug was shown to have effectiveness in the treatment of Parkinson's disease and was associated with a low incidence of side effects. While the patch is certainly useful and obviates taking drugs orally, some patients did suffer skin complications related to patch placement. However, the technology of patch therapy is rapidly advancing, and in the future there will certainly be some formulation of patch available for the treatment of Parkinson's disease.

COMT Inhibitors

A new class of drugs that has been recently introduced for the treatment of Parkinson's disease is the COMT inhibitor. One such drug is entacapone, which inhibits the enzyme COMT that is responsible, in part, for the metabolism of levodopa. Sinemet is a combination of two compounds, carbidopa and levodopa. The carbidopa blocks one enzyme responsible for the degradation of levodopa. Similarly, COMT inhibitors block another enzyme responsible for levodopa degradation. This results in increased blood levels of levodopa and subsequently increased levels of dopamine in the brain. These drugs have been conclusively shown to increase "on" time and decrease "off" time in patients with motor fluctuations. Other advantages of COMT inhibitors include immediate clinical response and reduction of the dose of levodopa by an average of 25 percent. Side effects of these drugs include dyskinesias, which can be managed by reducing levodopa dosage, and occasionally diarrhea, which in a few patients is severe enough to result in discontinuation of the drug.

COMT inhibitors are often used successfully in advanced disease and for patients with motor fluctuations. There are currently studies in progress looking at whether these drugs are useful in early disease. One theory is that constant stimulation of dopamine receptors and stable plasma levodopa levels will result in less motor fluctuation.

Other Drugs Under Investigation

A promising class of drugs currently being studied in animals is referred to as neurotrophic factors. These compounds appear to have the ability to revive dying cells and to rescue sick cells. Experiments in monkeys with these compounds have indeed been very encouraging. One injection of neurotrophic factors such as GDNF has caused reversal of parkinsonian symptoms. These compounds unfortunately cannot be given orally because they would not get in the brain. There is an ongoing investigation of GDNF in Parkinson's disease in which GDNF is put directly into a cavity of the brain called a ventricule by a surgical procedure. Results of these experiments are not yet known. There are also certain compounds called immunophylins that can be taken orally; these neurotrophic compounds are currently being studied in animals, and one of the agents in this class will most likely be available to study in humans. This is indeed a promising area of research in Parkinson's disease.

Another interesting class of drugs has been called glutamate antagonists. Glutamate, like dopamine, is a transmitter in the nervous system. It is referred to as an excitatory transmitter; data exists that if the nervous system becomes overactive (excess excitation), it may actually destroy neurons. The structure subthalamus in the basal ganglia uses the neurotransmitter glutamine; there is also glutamine transmission from the cerebral cortex to the striatum. Therefore, glutamine is clearly an important chemical related to Parkinson's disease. Currently drugs are being studied in Parkinson's disease that have the ability to block glutamine transmission. These drugs are being studied both as neuroprotective and symptomatic therapy, as well as antidyskinetic treatment. Riluzole is one drug in this class that is currently undergoing clinical trials, and patients at appropriate centers can volunteer for these studies.

Dopamine transport inhibitors are another class of drugs that can block the mechanism that turns off the effect of dopamine in the brain. The main way dopamine action is stopped in the brain is by reuptake into the presynaptic terminal. Drugs like cocaine and amphetamine work in part by blocking the dopamine transporter. Animals that have the dopamine transporter deleted genetically become exceedingly hyperactive. Increased excitation and insomnia are possible side effects of this class of drugs. Nevertheless, this approach represents a novel mechanism at attempting to increase dopamine in the brain.

There are also other drugs of possible benefit to Parkinson's patients that are currently undergoing study in the laboratory, but at this time there is not enough information to discuss these potential agents.

SURGICAL TREATMENT

There is also a variety of surgical treatments being used in the investigation of Parkinson's disease therapy, including neurotransplant, ablative lesions, and deep brain stimulation (DBS).

Studies of neuroplantation in Parkinson's disease have been conducted for several years. This approach is perhaps the most direct, involving placing new cells in the brain to replace the cells that are injured. Current cell sources that have been used include embryonic human tissue and, more recently, embryonic pig tissue. Results from these studies to date show a modest improvement which takes several months to develop. There is much ongoing research in this area. These studies are trying to determine the best way to optimize this form of therapy. Several autopsy reports from patients who received neurotransplants have shown that the cells which they received were not rejected, but instead were accepted by the brain and produced both increased neuronal activity and dopamine levels. It is clear that neurotransplant remains an exciting potential avenue of treatment. It is thought that cell sources other than human tissue will be needed to make this approach a more viable one.

The use of pallidotomy in the treatment of Parkinson's disease has gained increasing use worldwide. In this procedure, a lesion is put into a part of the brain called the globus pallidus. It is thought that this area is hyperactive because of the loss of dopamine in the nigro-striatal pathway. Recent research indicates that the symptom best treated with this procedure is dyskinesia on the opposite side of the body from the lesion. It is estimated that the mean decrease of dyskinesia is approximately 80 percent. Some patients have a total resolution of their other dyskinesias. Other Parkinson's disease symptoms such as tremor, rigidity, and bradykinesia are improved in the range of 25 to 30 percent. This is a moderate improvement; however, for some patients this will result in increased functional capabilities. Other symptoms that are difficult to treat with levodopa—such as freezing, low voice, and postural instability that leads to falling—do not respond well to pallidotomy. If these are the main problems that need to be corrected, the patient should not undergo pallidotomy. It has also become clear in recent years that bilateral pallidotomy (done on both sides of the brain to affect both sides of the body) may be associated with an unacceptable risk. Cognitive decline, speech abnormalities, and swallowing problems occur with a relatively high frequency in patients receiving bilateral pallidotomies, and as a result most centers will not perform the operation bilaterally. Nonetheless, the introduction of pallidotomy for advanced Parkinson's disease has helped many patients and is clearly an advance in our total management of Parkinson's disease.

Another innovative surgical approach is deep brain stimulation (DBS). This procedure is currently approved for unilateral treatment of Parkinson's disease tremor. With DBS, there is placement of an electrode in the brain area of the thalamus called the VIM nucleus. DBS of the VIM nucleus has been shown to be very effective in reducing parkinsonian tremor, but not the other symptoms of Parkinson's disease. The DBS electrode is implanted in the brain, which is connected by an extension wire to a pacemaker-like battery source called an impulse generator. It is thought that the high-frequency stimulation causes a block in this area of the brain. DBS has the advantage of not destroying part of the brain and therefore is reversible. It is also adaptable in that one can change the stimulus parameters to increase the effectiveness of the stimulus; likewise, one can decrease stimulation if adverse reactions occur. It also appears that bilateral operations can be done with this procedure with less long-term side effects. There is a 1 percent chance of intracerebral hemorrhage with this type of procedure. Adverse reactions can also occur related to the stimulation, although these are usually mild or related to the device itself, such as infection at the site.

Attempts are also being made to place the electrode for deep brain stimulation in other areas of the brain, particularly the globus pallidus and the subthalamus (STN). The placement of electrodes in these areas is particularly exciting as it appears that almost all symptoms of Parkinson's disease—not only tremor, but also bradykinesia, rigidity, levodopa-induced dyskinesias, freezing, postural instability, and gait—may be improved by this procedure. Initial results with STN stimulation appear very encouraging. Some patients have stopped their medication after effective DBS of the subthalamus. Currently these procedures are reserved for patients with advanced disease in which drugs no longer provide control of symptoms and quality of life has been markedly diminished. It is encouraging, however, that some patients receiving DBS have done particularly well. This is clearly a very promising area of research.

CONCLUSION

Patients should take heart at the depth and breadth of scientific research that is currently underway in Parkinson's disease. Everywhere in the world, doctors and scientists are studying either basic or clinical mechanisms that are related to Parkinson's disease. The major pharmaceutical companies are engaged in searching for better drugs for the treatment of this disorder. Clearly, research holds the key to our understanding of Parkinson's disease and the hope of eventually erasing this disorder from the world. Patients can play a major role in research in Parkinson's disease by volunteering for clinical trials. It is my opinion that scientists working with clinicians will be able to find the causes of and cure for Parkinson's disease in the near future.

Appendix A

Home Exercise Program

STRETCHING EXERCISES

These exercises help loosen up your tight muscles to improve your walking pattern. Do these exercises daily. Hold each stretch 20 to 30 seconds. Repeat 1 to 3 times.

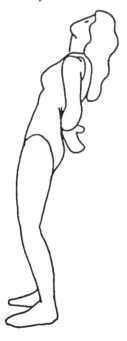

1. *Trunk bending forward and back:* Stand with feet flat on the floor. (Use a supportive surface if necessary.) Slowly bend at the waist trying to reach for the floor.

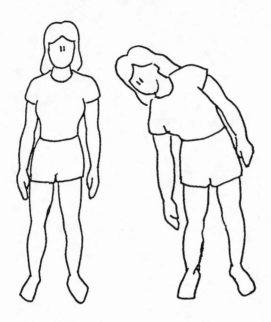

2. *Trunk bending side to side:* Same position as above in sitting or standing. With arms at your side, bend slowly at the waist to the right, then back to neutral. Then bend slowly to the left and back to neutral again.

3. *Trunk twists:* Same position as above in sitting or standing. Place hands at your waist and slowly twist to the right and then to the left.

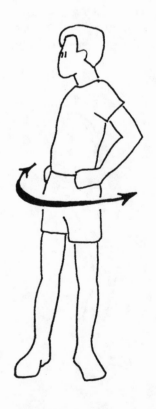

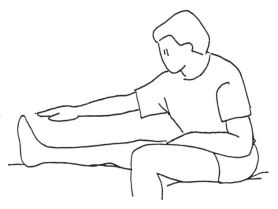

4. *Hamstring stretch:* Sitting, raise one leg up onto another chair. Point toes up and keep knee straight. Then try to reach toes.

RANGE OF MOTION (ROM) EXERCISES:

These exercises can be done actively, meaning without any resistance to movement. They can also be performed with resistance or cuff weights for strengthening or Progressive Resistance Exercises (PREs). These exercises help maintain ROM and strengthen arms and legs to enhance posture, transfers, balance, and walking. Do these exercises daily.

Standing Position

5. *Stepping up and down:* Face the step squarely and use a stable surface for support. Step up and down, concentrating on foot placement. Exchange the leading leg. Repeat 10 times.

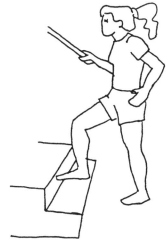

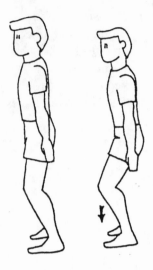

6. *Mini-squats:* Stand straight with feet a shoulder-width apart and arms at your sides. (Use a stable surface like a chair or countertop for extra support if needed.) Maintain your balance while bending knees. Keep feet flat on the floor with your back straight. Hold 5 seconds. Repeat 10 times.

7. *Marching in place:* Stand straight with feet a shoulder-width apart and arms at your sides. Hold onto a stable surface and alternately raise each knee to hip level, then lower it. Repeat 10 times.

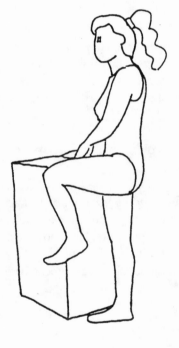

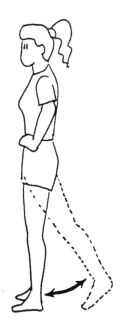

8. *Leg kicks to the back:* Stand straight with feet a shoulder-width apart and arms at your sides. Keep your body and knees straight. Slowly raise or extend one leg as far back as you can. Then slowly return to the starting position. Repeat 10 times on each leg.

9. *Leg kicks to the side:* Stand straight with feet a shoulder-width apart and arms at your sides. Keep your back and knees straight. Raise one leg to the side as far as you can. Then slowly return to the starting position. Repeat 10 times on each leg.

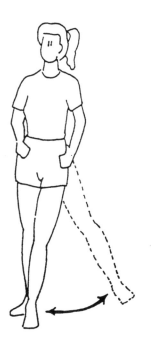

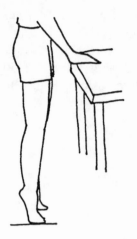 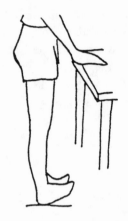

10. *Heel-toe raises:* Stand straight with feet a shoulder-width apart and arms at your sides. Gently rise up on the front half of the foot or toes. Then slowly roll back onto your heels with toes raised off the floor. Repeat 10 times.

11. *Heelcord stretch:* Stand with feet flat on the floor and a shoulder-width apart. Hold onto a stable surface and step one foot behind the other. Shift your weight forward over the front leg while keeping the back heel flat on the floor.

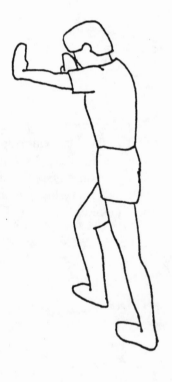

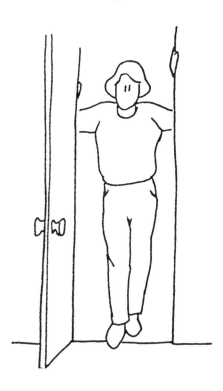

12. *Chest stretch:* With hands out to either side and facing forward against door facing, gently lean forward. Hold the position for 20 to 30 seconds. Repeat 1 to 3 times.

13. *Arm circles:* Swing your arms in a large forward circle 10 times. Then reverse direction and circle 10 times. Next make 10 small forward circles with arms out to the side. Then reverse direction and repeat small circles 10 times.

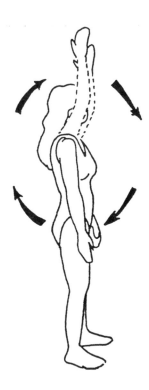

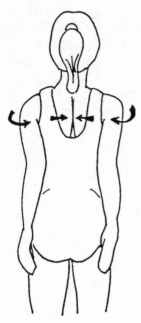

14. *Shoulder blade pinch:* Pull shoulders back, pinching shoulder blades together with arms at your sides. Hold 5 seconds. Repeat 10 times.

SITTING POSITION

15. *Ankle pumps:* Point toes up toward the ceiling and then point toes straight. Repeat 10 to 20 times.

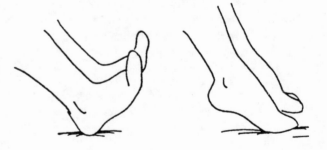

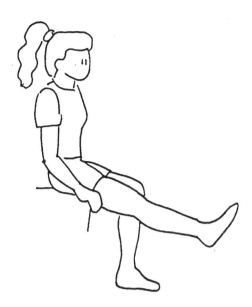

16. *Leg kicks:* Sit with your back straight and feet flat on the floor. Raise one leg up to straighten the knee. Hold the leg straight for 5 seconds and then slowly lower the leg. Repeat 10 times with each leg.

17. *Marching in place:* Sit with your back straight and feet flat on the floor. Alternately bend your hip and raise one foot off the floor. Repeat 10 to 20 times.

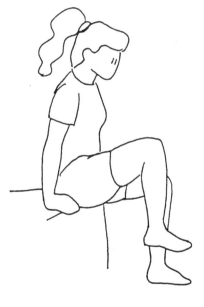

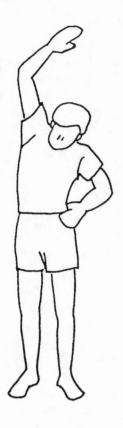

18. *Arm lifts:* Clasp hands together. Lift hands toward the ceiling. Hold 20 to 30 seconds. Repeat 3 times.

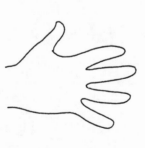

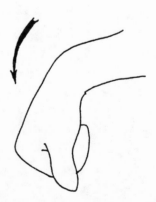

19. *Wrist and hand stretch:* Open hands as wide as you can and pull hand back, bending at the wrist. Hold 20 to 30 seconds. Then make a tight fist, rolling the fist down again and bending your wrist. Repeat 3 times.

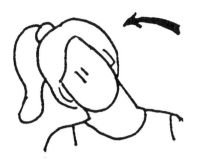

20. *Lateral neck stretch:* Gently tilt head to one side as far as possible. Hold 20 to 30 seconds. Repeat 3 times on each side.

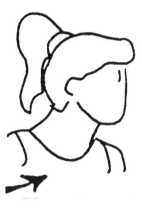

21. *Neck rotation:* Turn your head as far as possible to look over one shoulder. Hold 20 to 30 seconds. Repeat 3 times in each direction.

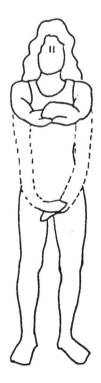

22. *Upper back stretch:* Stand or sit with chin tucked down and clasp hands in front of body. Extend arms forward while maintaining your back against the chair. Feel back muscles around shoulder blades stretch. Hold each position 20 to 30 seconds. Repeat 3 times.

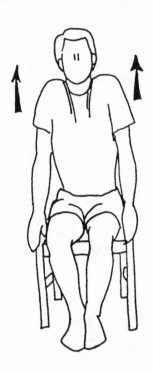

23. *Shoulder shrugs:* Raise shoulders toward your ears. Then drop shoulders down, stretching hands toward the floor. Repeat 10 times slowly.

MAT EXERCISES

These exercises are done lying on your back. Do these exercises one leg at a time.

24. *Heel slides:* Start with legs straight and relax. Bend at the knee and hip to slide one heel toward your buttocks. Slowly return to a straight position. Repeat 10 times with each leg.

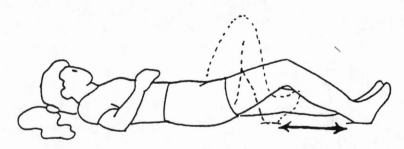

25. *Straight leg raises:* Bend one leg to support your back. Keep the other knee straight by tightening the muscles on top of your thigh. Gently raise the straight leg off the bed 4 to 6 inches. Slowly return to the starting position. Repeat 10 times with each leg.

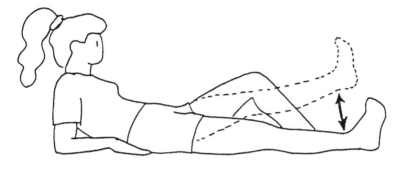

26. *Legs to the side:* Keep your legs and back straight. Move one leg out to the side while keeping the knee straight. Slowly return to the starting position. Repeat 10 times with each leg.

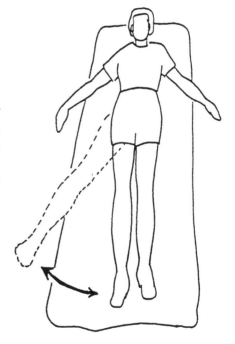

27. *Single knee to chest:* Lay on your back with knees bent. Grasp one knee and pull it toward your chest. Continue to breath slowly and deeply. Hold the stretch for 20 to 30 seconds. Slowly return to the starting position. Repeat 3 times with each leg.

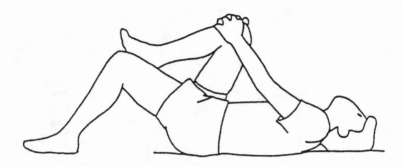

28. *Bridging:* Lie on back with knees bent, feet flat on the mat, and arms at sides. Raise hips off the mat and hold for 5 seconds. Slowly lower hips back to mat. Repeat 10 times.

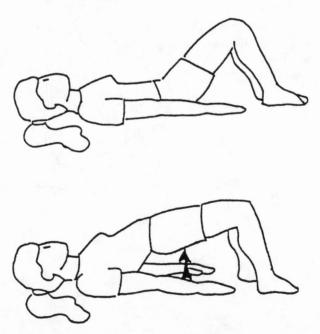

29. *Lower trunk rotation:* Lie on back with knees bent. Keep shoulders flat on the mat. Slowly roll knees over to the right side as far as possible and hold for 20 to 30 seconds. Repeat 3 times to each side.

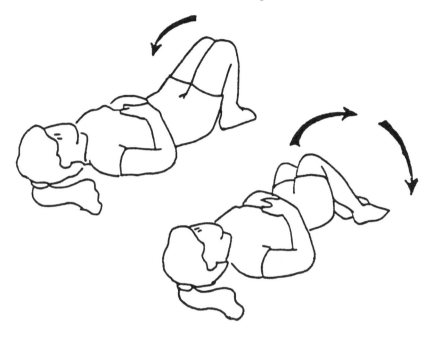

These exercises are done lying on your stomach.

30. *Elbow prop:* While lying on your stomach, prop your upper body up on your elbows. Hold for 10 seconds and relax. Repeat 10 times.

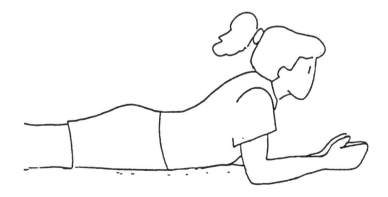

31. *Leg lifts:* Lie on your stomach with a pillow under your hips and resting your head on arms. Slowly raise one leg off of mat and hold 5 seconds, then slowly lower back to mat. Repeat 10 times with each leg.

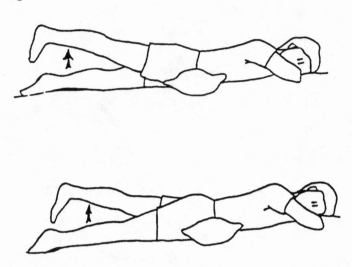

32. *Arm lifts:* Lie on your stomach with a pillow under your hips and your arms extended on either side of head. Slowly raise one arm off of mat and hold 5 seconds, then slowly lower back to mat. Repeat 10 times with each arm.

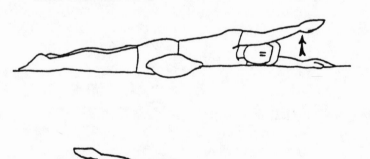

Glossary

Acetylcholine: one of the major chemicals in the brain, a neurotransmitter that stimulates motor nerves (see **Neurotransmitter**).

Action tremor: tremor that increases with voluntary movement.

Agonist: a class of drug which stimulates the dopamine receptors directly, thus increasing neurotransmitter activity.

Agnosia: inability to hear, see, or perceive even though the sensory systems are functioning and intact.

Akinesia: complete or partial loss of muscle movement.

Amantadine (hydrochloride): a medication initially designed to relieve influenza symptoms but later found to help rigidity, slowness of movement, and tremor in parkinsonism.

Amplification system: device to increase the loudness of speech.

Anticholinergic agents: substances (medications) that adversely affect nerve endings that allow the chemical acetylcholine to be emitted.

Antidepressant (medication): medications used to treat depression.

Antihistaminic medication: drugs designed to reduce the natural histamine level, which increases when certain tissues of the body are injured or irritated; they appear to have other properties that inhibit production of acetylcholine.

Antioxidant: agent that prevents the loss of oxygen (oxidation) in chemical reactions.

Antipsychotic (medication): medication used to treat psychosis.

Aphasia: inability to express oneself through speech.

Apraxia: inability to act in a purposeful way even though capable of moving and comprehending.

Arteriosclerotic: resulting from hardened arteries.

Aspiration: oral secretions, food, or liquids going into the airway.

Aspiration pneumonia: pneumonia that occurs after having breathed foreign matter into the lungs.

Autonomic nervous system: nervous system that serves the involuntary body functions (e.g., breathing, the beating of the heart).

Basal ganglia: clusters of cells located deep in the brain and crucial for coordinating motor commands.

Benzodiazepine: a class of tranquilizers, which includes diazepam (Valium), chlordiazepoxide (Librium), and alprazolam (Xanax), which do not result in parkinsonism or Parkinson-like symptoms.

Bilateral: occurring on both sides of the body (left and right).

Biofeedback: a behavior modification in which patients are taught to partially control unconscious bodily functions, such as bood pressure and heart rate.

Blepharospasm: rapid blinking or forced closure of the eyes.

Blood pressure cuff: the part of the instrument used for measuring blood pressure that is wrapped around the upper arm.

Bradykinesia: slow or reduced movement.

Bradyphrenia: slow thinking.

Center of gravity: the point at which the pull of gravity of any mass is centered.

Central nervous system: the brain and spinal cord.

Carbidopa (Lodosyn): a drug used in combination with levodopa in the treatment of Parkinson's disease which prevents levodopa from being metabolized in the body, thus allowing more levodopa to reach the brain.

Chlorpromazine (Thorazine): a tranquilizing medication that can cause Parkinson-like symptoms.

Cholinergic system: system of nerve endings that permit the emission of the chemical acetylcholine.

ChriCadence: rhythm of measured movement.

Clonazepam: medication to relieve sudden muscle spasms (see **Nocturnal myoclonus**).

Cognition: awareness; having perception and memory.

Cogwheeling: refers to increased muscular tone (stiffness) of Parkinson's disease; the increased tone, when felt by the examiner, produces regular jerks like pulling on a cogwheel.

Cohesive: to stick or hold together.

Condom catheter: a condom-like apparatus that fits over the penis in a manner that permits emptying of the bladder into a bag connected to the catheter with tubing.

Constipation: a change in the frequency and/or the consistency of bowel movements.

Corpus striatum: a vital part of the brain, located beneath the cerebral cortex (outer covering of the brain) and comprised of two basal ganglia (caudate and putamen).

Chorea: rapid, jerky, dance-like movements of the body.

Cortex: the outer layer of the cerebrum, densely packed with nerve cells.

Cyclotron: instrument used to smash electrons, thereby emitting energy for analysis.

Delirium: disorientation with respect to time and place, often accompanied by illusions and hallucinations; a state of mental confusion/excitement.

Dementia: progressive deterioration of mental state.

Demerol: an addictive pain medication.

Dehydration: condition resulting from an excessive loss of body fluids.

Distended abdomen: stretched or inflated abdomen.

Dopa decarboxylase: an enzyme in the body that converts levodopa to dopamine.

Dopa decarboxylase inhibitors: antiparkinson drugs that block the dopa decarboxylase enzyme and stop levadopa from changing into dopamine in the peripheral circulation, thus allowing more levadopa to go to the brain.

Dopamine: a chemical produced by the brain; it assists in the effective transmission of electrochemical messages between neurons (see **Neurotransmitter**).

Dopaminergic: a chemical that works like dopamine or has the same effect as dopamine.

Dyskinesia: abnormal, involuntary movement of voluntary muscles (e.g., in the hand, arm, leg, etc.) including twitches, jerks, twisting, or writhing movements.

Dysphagia: difficulty swallowing.

Dystonia: slow, twisting movements which may involve one limb or almost the entire body.

Encephalitis: inflammation of the brain.

Endocrine disorders: diseases or dysfunctions of any or all of the following glandular network: thyroid, parathyroid, adrenal gland, pituitary (anterior and posterior), testes/ovaries.

Enzyme: a substance that speeds up a chemical reaction but is not consumed in the reaction itself.

Essential tremor: a rapid tremor that, in contrast to the slower, resting tremor of Parkinson's disease, increases with limb extension (see **Tremor**).

Esophagus: body structure that connects the throat to the stomach and which food and liquid pass through.

Familial tremor: an inherited essential tremor (see **Tremor**).

Fecal impaction: feces wedged in the bowel, making elimination very difficult.

Festinating gait: rapid, uncontrolled shuffling.

Flexion: a joint in its bent position.

Flexion contracture: permanent bending of parts of the body.

Fluphenazine (Prolixin): a tranquilizing medication that can cause Parkinson-like symptoms.

Freezing: temporary, involuntary inability to move.

Gastric motility: speed at which the food you ingest moves through the gastrointestinal system.

Glaucoma: increased pressure of the eyeball, which can result in nerve damage and blindness.

Gray matter: a description of the outermost layer of the brain; the cortical tissue of the brain where thinking and information processing occur. This wrinkled surface of the brain is called the *cerebral cortex*.

Haloperidol (Haldol): a tranquilizing medication that can cause Parkinson-like symptoms.

Heimlich maneuver: a form of first aid for choking victims.

Hypomanic mood: mild excitement with moderate change in behavior.

Idiopathic: of unknown cause.

Incontinence: involuntary voiding of the bladder or bowel.

Impotence: the inability to achieve and/or maintain an erection.

Infused (intravenous): introducing a substance to the body via injection through a vein.

Intelligibility: level of understandable speech.

Lacunes: small strokes.

Loxapine (Loxitane): a tranquilizing medication that can cause Parkinson-like symptoms.

Levodopa: antiparkinson drug which is changed into dopamine in the brain; usually combined with carbidopa.

Levodopa "honeymoon": a period of time after treatment with levodopa begins when Parkinson's disease symptoms seem very slight or nonexistent.

Metabolism: the assimilation and processing of substances in the body (e.g., transforming food into energy, utilizing vitamin and mineral compounds, etc.).

Micrographia: small handwriting; in Parkinson's disease, writing may start out normal size and become smaller and smaller. Sometimes an early symptom of Parkinson's disease.

Monoamine oxidase (MAO): an enzyme that breaks down dopamine. Two types are MAO A and MAO B. In Parkinson's disease it is beneficial to block MAO B enzymes.

Motor diaries: a record of the level of motor function during a 24-hour period kept by recording sleep time, "on" time, and/or "off" time.

Motor performance: ability and capacity to move about and to maneuver the body.

MPTP (N-methyl-4-phenyl-1,2,3,6-tetrahydropyridine): a toxic chemical, the use of which can lead to parkinsonism.

Multi-infarct: interruption of blood flow, which results in strokes.

Muscle atrophy: wasting of muscle tissue due to lack of use as a result of being immobilized or from injury to the nerve that normally stimulates a muscle.

Musculoskeletal: the interrelationship of muscles and bone structures.

Neurofibrillary tangles: tangles of tiny fibers in nerve cells.

Neuron: a nerve cell.

Neurotransmitter: chemicals that permit nerve cell communication in the brain.

Neurovegetative syndrome: a state of altered awareness and reduced mental functioning with intact digestive, excretory, and other bodily processes.

Nocturnal myoclonus: sudden muscle jerks occurring at night.

Norepinephrine: a hormone secreted by the adrenal medulla and elsewhere; a neurotransmitter.

Off dystonia: an abnormal posturing or cramping when levodopa levels are at their minimum in the bloodstream (see **Levodopa**).

"Off" time: time during which antiparkinsonian medications are not working well and motor function is poor.

Oil retention enema: oil injected into the rectum to soften feces to improve elimination.

On dystonia (dyskinesia): abnormal movement when levodopa levels are at their peak in the bloodstream (usually 20 to 60 minutes after dosage).

"On" time: time during which antiparkinsonian medications are working well and motor function is good.

On-off fluctuation: fluctuations in response to antiparkinsonian drugs in which patient changes suddenly from a good response—"on"—to a poor response—"off."

Orthostatic hypotension: a drop in blood pressure during rapid changes in body position (e.g., from a sitting position to standing position).

Palsy: paralysis of a muscle or group of muscles.

Paroxysmal disorder: sudden onset of a disease or symptom.

Peak-dose dyskinesia: a type of dyskinesia which occurs when the dopamine in the brain is supposed to be at its peak; results from too much dopamine in the system.

Perseveration: repeating meaningless statements, phrases, or words or speaking repetitively when it bears no relation to the context.

Postencephalitic parkinsonism: parkinsonism that results from inflammation and infection of the brain.

Preclinical: prior to diagnosis of a disease.

Propulsive gait: walking that is propelled forward.

Psychomotor agitation: physical activity due to excited state of mind.

Psychotic disorder: mental disturbance resulting in loss of personality and loss of contact with reality.

Pulmonary emboli: a mass of undissolved matter in the main artery of the lung or one of its branches.

Radio labeled: marking a substance for detection with radiation.

Range of motion: the extent that a joint will move from full extension or full flexion.

Reserpine: a drug prescribed for high blood pressure or as a tranquilizer; its use may give rise to parkinsonism.

Resting tremor: shaking even though the body (or limb) is not being put in motion by the effected individual (see **Tremor**).

Retropulsive gait: walking that is propelled backward.

Rigidity: increased resistance to passive movement of a limb.

SSRIs (specific serotonin re-uptake inhibitors): a class of antidepressant medications.

Serotonin: neurotransmitter important in sleep and sensory perception.

Sialorrhea: drooling.

SLP (speech-language pathologist): an individual with a graduate degree who evaluates and treats communication disorders. Sometimes referred to as a "speech therapist."

Substantial nigra: an area of the midbrain containing a cluster of black-pigmented nerve cells that produce dopamine.

Toxin: a poisonous substance.

Tremor: rhythmic shaking; an involuntary movement of part(s) of the body as a result of sequential muscle contractions.

Tremulous voice: trembling or shaking voice.

Trifluroperazine (Stelazine): a tranquilizing medication that can cause Parkinson-like symptoms.

Voice inflection: change of pitch or tone.

Wearing off: a fluctuation in response to antiparkinsonian medications when the medications are losing their effect and marked parkinsonian symptoms progressively appear. Medication effects end before the next dose is due.

Author Profiles

Britt Allen, M.S., P.T., is a practicing physical therapist and active Center Administrator of Lubbock Rehability facilities. He received his B.S. in Physical Therapy in 1993 and M.S. in Interdisciplinary Studies in 1997. He was original physical therapist for the Parkinson Outreach multi-therapy rehabilitation program in Lubbock, Texas.

Angela R. Bednarz, R.N., B.S.N., is a Clinical Research Coordinator at the Neurology Research and Education Center, an affiliate of Covenant Health System in Lubbock, Texas. A research coordinator since 1992, she has experience in conducting clinical trials for new medications to treat Parkinson's disease and Alzheimer's disease. She also presents lectures and continuing education programs to health care personnel, patients, and family members on Parkinson's disease and Alzheimer's disease.

Kristi F. Bennett is the lead occupational therapist with the Parkinson's Outreach Program in Lubbock, Texas. She has developed several therapy programs in conjunction with the Parkinson Outreach Program and has presented lectures on "Rehabilitation for Parkinson's Disease." She is also the lead occupational therapist in the Neurological Rehabilitation Department at the Rehability Center in Lubbock, Texas.

Joan I. Dickinson, M.S., is a doctoral student and graduate instructor in the Department of Merchandising, Environmental Design and Consumer Economics at Texas Tech University in Lubbock. She is the author of "Wandering Behavior and Attempted Exits Among Residents Diagnosed with Dementia-Related Illnesses: A Qualitative Approach," *Journal of Women and Aging* (1998), "Wandering Behavior Associated with Alzheimer's Disease and Related Dementias: Implications for Designers," *Journal of Interior Design* (1996), and "The Effects of Visual Barriers on Exiting Behavior in Dementia Care Unit," *The Gerontologist* (1995).

Bhupesh H. Dihenia, M.D., is in the private practice of neurology and is a research scientist with the Neurology Research and Education Center at Covenant Health System in Lubbock, Texas. Dr. Dihenia did his neurology residency at Emory University, where he also completed a fellowship in sleep disorders and movement disorders. Part of his training included working with the neurological team developing microelectode monitoring for pallidotomy surgery at Emory University.

Raye Lynne Dippel, Ph.D., is a clinical and lifespan developmental psychologist in private practice in Colorado Springs, Colorado. She was formerly assistant professor in the Department of Psychiatry at the University of Texas Medical School in Houston and in the Department of Psychology at Lamar University in Beaumont, Texas. Dr. Dippel is co-editor with J. Thomas Hutton of *Caring for the Parkinson Patient: A Practical Guide* and *Caring for the Alzheimer's Patient: A Practical Guide.*

J. Thomas Hutton, M.D., Ph.D., is the director of the Neurology Research and Education Center and medical director of the National Parkinson Foundation Center of Excellence at Covenant Health System in Lubbock, Texas. He is a clinical professor in the Department of Neuropsychiatry and Behavioral Sciences at Texas Tech University Health Sciences Center. As a practicing neurologist, he carries out an active research program in Parkinson's disease. He is the author of over 100 articles and six books and chapters on Parkinson's disease, Alzheimer's disease, and related disorders. He is the past president of the Texas Neurological Society.

Trudy Hutton, J.D., is administrator of the Neurology Research and Education Center and patient services coordinator of the National Parkinson Foundation Center of Excellence at Covenant Health System in Lubbock, Texas. As an attorney, she specializes in family law. Ms. Hutton has long experience in education working with patients and their families suffering from neurological diseases. She edits a newsletter for Parkinson's disease patients and their families and lectures about caregiver issues to support groups. She has written a number of articles about the practical aspects of coping with Parkinson's disease for patients.

Jeffrey W. Elias, Ph.D., is professor and associate chair of the Department of Psychology at Texas Tech University in Lubbock, Texas. His research program has concentrated on the cognitive changes that occur with age and the effects of disease processes on normal aging. Dr. Elias is the experimental studies editor of *Experimental Aging Research.* He is also coeditor of the text *Cardiovascular Disease and Behavior.*

Susan Imke, R.N., M.S., is a certified family nurse practitioner and serves as Director of Patient Services for the National Parkinson Foundation. She has extensive experience working with older adults who are coping with chronic health problems and is actively involved in clinical practice, research, and educational programs for caregivers as well as health care professionals interested in Parkinson's disease and Alzheimer's disease.

William C. Koller, M.D., Ph.D., is professor and chairman of the Department of Neurology at the University of Kansas Medical Center in Kansas City. Dr. Koller is interested in research in Parkinson's disease and tremor disorders. He is Chairman of the International Tremor Foundation. He is actively involved in research in Parkinson's disease and is the editor of *Handbook of Parkinson's Disease*, the coeditor of *Therapeutic Approaches to Parkinson's Disease,* and the author of numerous articles related to movement disorders.

Matthew E. Lambert, Ph.D., is in the private practice of neuropsychology. He is a research associate with the Neurology Research and Education Center at Covenant Health System in Lubbock, Texas. Dr. Lambert has developed programs for dealing with anxiety and panic in Parkinson's disease.

Terry C. McMahon, M.D., is an associate professor of psychiatry and assistant dean for medical education in the School of Medicine at the Texas Tech University Health Sciences Center in Lubbock, Texas. As director of the Psychiatric Consultation Liaison Service and director of Undergraduate Education in Psychiatry, he has played an active role in developing clinical lectures and seminars for medical students and residents in geriatric psychiatry.

Jerry L. Morris, M.A., is a research associate at the Neurology Research and Education Center in Lubbock, Texas. He has worked in Parkinson's disease and Alzheimer's disease research for approximately 12 years. He has coordinated clinical drug trials and basic research studies, as well as coauthored numerous articles and book chapters.

Janet Schwantz, M.S., CCC/SP, has been a speech-language pathologist since receiving her master's degree in 1982 from the University of North Texas. She currently practices at the Neurology Research and Education Center, a National Parkinson Foundation Center of Excellence at Covenant Health System in Lubbock, Texas, where she is coordinator of the Parkinson's Disease Speech Therapy Program. She is involved in the research of speech, swallowing, and communication problems of Parkinson's disease patients. Ms. Schwantz lectures on speech, swallowing, and communication problems of Parkinson's disease patients and supervises graduate speech pathology students for Texas Tech University and for Texas Women's University.

Lauren Seeberger, M.D., is the medical co-director of the Colorado Neurological Institute Movement Disorders Center, a National Parkinson Foundation Center of Excellence, in Denver. She serves as medical advisor to the Parkinson's Association of the Rockies. Dr. Seeberger is a member of the Parkinson's Study Group and is active in clinical research in Parkinson's disease.

JoAnn Shroyer, Ph.D., is a professor in the area of environmental design at Texas Tech University and serves as an associate research scientist at the Neurology Research and Education Center at Covenant Health System, Lubbock, Texas. She is also Executive Director of the Retired Senior Volunteer Program, Lubbock, Texas, and chair of the Department of Merchandising, Environmental Design and Consumer Economics. She has been a faculty member at Texas Tech University since 1984. Dr. Shroyer received her doctorate from Oklahoma State University in housing, design, and consumer studies with a collateral in gerontology. Her research, teaching, and service has been recognized with awards, including the President's Excellence in Teaching Award at Texas Tech University and the Environmental Design Research Award from the American Society of Interior Designers. She conducts research in the area of environmental design needs for individuals with Alzheimer's disease and Parkinson's disease. She presented over 50 papers at international, national, and state professional meetings. In addition, she has published over 30 articles, chapters, books, and technical monographs. Among her research interests is the assessment of environmental design factors that contribute to falling among those with Parkinson's disease.

Janice M. Stewart, R.N., B.S.N., is a Clinical Research Coordinator at the Neurology Research and Education Center at Covenant Health System in Lubbock, Texas. A research coordinator since 1992, she has experience in conducting clinical trials for new medications to treat Parkinson's disease and Alzheimer's disease. She also presents lectures and continuing education programs to health care personnel, patients, and family members on Parkinson's disease and Alzheimer's disease.

Ginah S. Vrooman, P.T., is the neurology department physical therapist of the Rehability Center in Lubbock, Texas. She has been practicing physical therapy since 1990. Ms. Vrooman specializes in adult and geriatric patients with neurological disorders. She is currently physical therapist for the Parkinson's Outreach Program.

Charles R. Walker, Ph.D., is a neuropsychologist and clinical psychologist currently in private practice in Lubbock, Texas. Dr. Walker has served as an assistant professor in Psychology and Rehabilitation Science at the University of Texas Southwestern Medical Center in Dallas. At Southwestern, he worked for several years at the Alzheimer's and Related Disorders Clinic. Dr. Walker is an adjunct assistant professor of psychology at Texas Tech University in Lubbock.

Karen Boyd Worley, Ph.D., is a psychologist and director of the Family Treatment Program at Arkansas Children's Hospital. She is assistant professor in the Department of Pediatrics at the University of Arkansas for Medical Sciences. Dr. Worley specializes in assessment and treatment of families in which sexual abuse has occurred. She is an experienced lecturer and has published several articles in the area of child abuse.